PSYCHOSOMATIC METHODS
IN PAINLESS CHILDBIRTH

TO
ODETTE AND PASCALE

PSYCHOSOMATIC METHODS IN PAINLESS CHILDBIRTH

History, Theory and Practice

by

L. CHERTOK

Médecin-Assistant du Centre de
Médecine Psychosomatique de Villejuif

with foreword by
Professor W. C. W. NIXON, M.D., F.R.C.S. F.R.C.O.G.

Translated from the 2nd French edition of
Les Méthodes Psychosomatiques d'Accouchement sans Douleur

by

DENIS LEIGH, M.D.

Also translated into Spanish and Italian

PERGAMON PRESS
LONDON - NEW YORK - PARIS - LOS ANGELES
1959

PERGAMON PRESS LTD.
4 & 5 Fitzroy Square, London W.1

PERGAMON PRESS INC.
122 East 55th Street, New York 22, N.Y.
P.O. Box 47715, Los Angeles, California

PERGAMON PRESS S.A.R.L.
24 Rue des Écoles, Paris V^e.

Copyright
©
1959
L. CHERTOK

Library of Congress Card No. 58-12663

Printed by J. W. Arrowsmith Ltd., in Great Britain

AUTHOR'S PREFACE TO THE 1st EDITION

THE nomenclature of the non-pharmacological methods of producing analgesia has always posed a problem. Read's method, first entitled 'natural childbirth', later became 'childbirth without fear'. The Russian method, originally christened 'psychoprophylaxis of the pains of childbirth', has recently become 'psychoprophylactic preparation of pregnant women for childbirth'. These methods, or their variants, have also gone under different names such as psychophysical, psychophysiotherapeutic or neurophysical methods, or yet again as childbirth without pain, without fear, without suffering, without anxiety, without apprehension, childbirth with diminished pain, and many others.

None of these expressions is entirely satisfactory. For instance, 'natural childbirth' is a misnomer, for the painless quality of natural childbirth is unproven. Neither does 'childbirth without fear' describe the facts, for the aim is not only to reduce the fear, but equally the pain. Even if the analgesia is not always complete, some degree of analgesia can nevertheless be attained.

As to the term psychoprophylactic, the effect on the pain is not always at a prophylactic, but may just as well be at a therapeutic, level. In addition, the term 'psychoprophylactic preparation of pregnant women for childbirth' fails to take into account that important part of the method which is concerned with the conduct to be observed during the birth itself. Nonetheless, it does not seem that these diverse phrases correspond to essential differences in the methods themselves. In each the important factor is the psychological, and on this account it seems reasonable to bring them together under the title of 'psychosomatic methods'.

For the last twenty years or so the term psychosomatic (although not entirely satisfactory owing to the dualism implicit in the word) has been used to describe a medicine in the Hippocratic tradition, which deals with man as a whole. Psychosomatic medicine implies a multiple causality, and emphasizes the role of psychological factors in man's biological functions. (12, 139) The pain of childbirth having psychological and physiological components, so therefore must the methods by which it is controlled be concerned with both aspects. However, the phrase 'painless childbirth' has been retained (although the result cannot always be considered in terms of the analgesia alone), chiefly because it is widely familiar to both the general public and the medical profession in France.

It is not proposed to question the efficacy of this or that method for it seems that good results can be obtained with all of them provided they are carried out under favourable conditions. Rather will they be described, and their theoretical bases discussed, separating off the scientific from what still remains hypothetical. By so doing, it will be possible to dispose of certain errors which are prejudicial to the methods, and to enable practitioners to act in a more rational manner.

Finally, I would like to thank Dr. Paul Walter for allowing me to work on his service at the Hôpital Rothschild. I was enabled to investigate the psychoprophylactic method and to make a pilot study of the different stages of the method by carrying out rapid or extemporary preparation in women who had not followed a regular preparation, including both normal and pathological pregnancies. The co-operation and understanding of the midwives and nursing staff in this work has been particularly appreciated.

January 1957.

AUTHOR'S PREFACE TO THE 2nd EDITION

The first edition of this book was exhausted one year after its publication. The attention it attracted may be considered as a sign of an increasing interest in painless childbirth. Following the initial period, marked at times by undue enthusiasm, or by equally exaggerated scepticism, non-pharmacological obstetrical analgesia now occupies its rightful place in medical practice.

Psychosomatic methods, moreover, encompass more than the field of analgesia alone, but bring obstetrical and medical advantages and, above all, open broad psychological and socia perspectives.

There undoubtedly remain many controversial points upon which investigations are attempting to shed new light.

A useful survey of opinion resulted from the symposium held in Paris, on 7 April 1957, and it has been valuable to report the main trends of the discussions which then took place. A critical analysis will also be made of the main publications which have appeared since the first edition appeared.

The chapter concerned with the Hypnosuggestive Method in Russia has been considerably extended and thoroughly revised. We do in fact, believe that the best understanding of the methods in use today can be gained by giving an account of what has preceded them. Thanks to the courtesy of the Medical Library in Moscow, we have received microfilms of very interesting publications unobtainable in France.

A chapter has been added on the collaboration of the husband, that concerning mental hygiene has been extended, and additions have been made to every chapter.

In the course of our personal investigations, we have come to inquire searchingly into some theoretical concepts and the results of our reflections will be given in a new chapter entitled 'Attempt at Formulation'.

We hope that the new material in this edition will prove of value to those who will use it and in this way the book may even better fulfil its role of informing practitioners and of inspiring them in their own studies. *January* 1958.

CONTENTS

Author's Prefaces		v, vii
Foreword		xi
Introduction		xiii
1. Analgesia and Psychotherapy		1
2. The First Obstetrical Analgesias produced by Hypnosuggestive Techniques		11
3. Hypnosuggestive Methods in Obstetrics at the End of the 19th Century		15
4. Evolution of the Conception of Hypnosis		19
5. Hypnosuggestive Methods in Germany and Austria after the First World War		23
6. Hypnosuggestive Methods in Russia after 1923		30
7. The Read Method		53
8. Hypnosuggestive Methods in Anglo-Saxon Countries after the Second World War		87
9. The Psychoprophylactic Method in the Soviet Union		92
10. The Application of the Psychoprophylactic Method in France and throughout the World		151
11. A Comparison of the Methods of Read and Velvovski		175
12. An Examination of the Problems		184
Conclusion		221
Bibliography		223
Name Index		253
Subject Index		258

FOREWORD

THE problem of pain in labour is one of great concern to any humane community. Approaches to it have varied at different times and places. Many contributions have been made during the last 100 years by the English-speaking countries but at the present time, curiously, doctors from these parts of the world lag behind their colleagues in other countries in their interest in what may broadly be termed psychosomatic preparation for childbirth; indeed they seem largely unaware how keenly the matter is being discussed and studied elsewhere. Stimulating as it is this debate has centred rather too much on the relative merits of different methods and has suffered, moreover, from the proponents of one method being insufficiently acquainted with other methods. This, together with the limitation of outlook that specialization often imposes, has delayed the understanding of the deeper processes involved. In this book a psychiatrist enters the field, one who has for long interested himself in liaison between psychiatry and other medical specialities and more recently has been particularly engaged in studying psychological analgesia in childbirth. His knowledge of languages has further equipped him to survey the subject exceptionally widely. He has presented many brilliant comparisons and observations which should stimulate readers to explore the subject more deeply for themselves. Indeed, many will be led to feel that we are only at the commencement of our discovery of the possibilities and implications of this whole matter and that attempted experiment and analysis have often been based on inadequate knowledge or appreciation of all that is involved.

Anyone who has the care of women during one of the most vital moments in their lives feels dissatisfied if he suspects he has done less than his best for them. He relies, very properly, chiefly on his own experience; but honest enquiry into the experiences of others sometimes surprises him by the possibilities it opens up or suggests. Dr. Chertok has greatly assisted such an enquiry both by gathering a wealth of evidence and by turning the reader's mind to the consideration of basic concepts. He has thereby rendered an invaluable service.

W. C. W. NIXON
Professor of Obstetrics and Gynecology,
University College Hospital, London.

INTRODUCTION

CHILDBIRTH is a psychosomatic process *par excellence*, the mental state playing an important part in its progression. Psychology and physiology are here indissolubly linked and both are equally concerned in the pain of childbirth. A constant struggle has been waged against this pain and against the other difficulties of childbirth. In primitive civilizations numerous magical procedures were and are used to facilitate labour. It was only towards the middle of the nineteenth century that drugs came into general use, drugs which were, however, not without danger to both mother and child. There has been a constant search for new methods of relieving pain, methods which, if possible, should be deprived of all toxicity.

In France at present a lively interest is being taken in this problem. In 1952, in Paris, LAMAZE and VELLAY [298] introduced, at the Polyclinique des Métallurgistes, the psychoprophylactic method which originated in the Soviet Union, and has been described by VELVOVSKI and his co-workers in 1949 [553]. Their example was followed in other maternity units in Paris and in the Provinces as well as outside France. This resurgence of interest in the lessening of the pain of childbirth by non-pharmacological methods has coincided in France with the renewal, by some workers, of research inspired by the work of Grantly Dick Read. Appearing in 1933, Read's studies have not previously been applied on a large scale.

Public interest has been aroused, as is shown by numerous popular publications, newspaper articles, programmes on radio and television, and at a different level, the Pope's message in 1956 to an International Assembly of Gynaecologists and Obstetricians [3].

On 7 April 1957, a symposium was held in Paris, organized by the French Society of Psychosomatic Medicine, devoted to Psychological Analgesia in Obstetrics. A group of obstetricians, neurologists, psychiatrists, psychoanalysts and psychologists from France, Belgium, Italy, Spain, Portugal and Switzerland also took part. Grantly Dick Read, the author of the book

Natural Childbirth, attended and Velvovski, the originator of the Psychoprophylactic Method, sent a communication. Out of this meeting grew a project to organize a World Conference in 1961 on this same subject. On 5 June 1957 a Symposium on Psychoprophylactic Childbirth, presided over by Grantly Dick Read, was held in Turin.

The World Congress of Obstetrics and Gynaecology which will take place in Montreal in June 1958 has chosen as one of its subjects the question of psychological analgesia in obstetrics. The majority of the National Societies for Obstetrics and Gynaecology in Europe and America have also held special sessions on this problem.

The practice of these methods has given interesting results, but their evaluation in quantitative terms is difficult owing to the lack of instruments which enable us to measure objectively the feeling of pain. Certainly one cannot speak of the abolition of the pain of childbirth; nevertheless the introduction of non-pharmacological methods of obstetrical analgesia has been an advance because it brings a humanization and a dedramatization to the act of childbirth. Doctors, midwives and nurses have become more interested in the pregnant woman.

Historically, it is to hypnosis that one turns to discover the first results of a non-pharmacological obstetrical analgesia, but hypnosuggestive methods were only practised episodically and on a very small scale. In 1933 Grantly Dick Read described his method of 'natural childbirth', simple to practise and capable of a widespread application. In fact, however, it only reached a very limited public. It is with the method developed by Velvovski that non-pharmacological analgesia became at last the object of a more general study and practice in Europe. On the other hand Read's method lately has tended to become more widely known in Europe and in the United States. From the practical point of view, whatever may be the differences, and these will be referred to later, between the method of Read and that of Velvovski, both consist of didactic, physiotherapeutic and psychotherapeutic*

---

*Velvovski uses the word psychoprophylactic, but it will be seen later on that it is difficult to establish the boundary between psychotherapy and psychoprophylaxis.

elements. From the theoretical point of view these methods have still no solid foundation, and a series of controversies has taken place on this subject in France, in the U.S.A. and in the Soviet Union. Numerous problems which have been posed still remain without a solution to the present day.

The principal question is this: what is the cause of the modification of pain perception? As to hypnosis this question is superfluous, analgesia by means of suggestion having been known for many years; however, with regard to the English and Russian methods, their proponents place a variable importance on educational, psychotherapeutic and physiotherapeutic factors. Later, during the course of the argument in this book, it will be shown that in reality these different factors are interrelated. Read himself considers that the fundamental cause of the pain of childbirth is fear. On this account his method largely consists in the suppression of this fear. According to NICOLAIEV, one of the originators and chief theoreticians of the psychoprophylactic methods, the 'primordial role in all the methods of obstetrical analgesia is played by the psychotherapeutic or psychoprophylactic component, which in its turn consists of two factors. (1) A verbal action directly on the pregnant or parturient woman and (2) a series of "organizational factors" which have an "indirect" psychotherapeutic influence on the woman' [392]. It may thus be seen that in the three methods we have mentioned, the principal role is played by psychological factors acting at a prophylactic or a therapeutic level. It still remains for us to explain the processes by which psychotherapy produces relief of pain. This is the chief problem. How does a psychological happening modify pain perception? This psychophysiological problem, a problem of consciousness, still remains very ill-understood. Both the physiological and psychological explanations remain extremely hypothetical.

In order to clarify these problems we believe it is useful to return to a consideration of the facts. For this purpose the history of psychologically induced analgesia by hypnosis will be discussed on account of its experimental interest. The suggestive practices which were popular in nineteenth-century France, following the First World war in Germany and in Austria, after 1923 in the Soviet Union, and since the last war in the Anglo-Saxon countries, will then be discussed. In these latter countries the interest in psychologically induced analgesia in obstetrics has been reawakened by the diffusion of the British method of Grantly Dick Read. The theoretical aspects of this method will be discussed before passing to its practice, but the latter will not be the primary object and will not be considered in great detail. Read's book *Childbirth Without Fear* should be read by those who require greater practical detail. The criticisms of the method will be reported, chiefly theoretical criticisms for which American writers are largely responsible. One chapter will be devoted to the combination of Read's method with the Autogenous Training developed by J. H. Schultz of Germany. The Psychoprophylactic Method as it is practised and conceived in the U.S.S.R. will also be considered in detail. Much work has already been carried out in France on the Russian method; the subject has been presented in a partial manner, and some of its aspects have been insufficiently emphasized. Its genesis and evolution require further consideration. In addition, the hypothetic character of the theoretical position was not always stressed, and thus the differences of opinion in the Soviet Union have been neglected. The applications of the Psychoprophylactic Method in France and other countries will be discussed in a later chapter. We shall make a comparative study of the English and Russian methods by considering criticism of the former by French and other authors. An attempt has been made to systematically discuss the principal problems concerning the following: pain in general, the pain of childbirth, psychologically induced analgesia, obstetrical analgesia, the participation of the husband, and the results of the treatment of pregnant women by these methods and lastly the whole problem of mental health. All these problems which bring out the relationships between psychology and physiology remain very much unanswered. However it is as well to state that the differences between the methods of painless childbirth are more apparent than real. All these methods in effect depend on the same principle, the same process, call it psychotherapeutic, psychoprophylactic or purely verbal.

CHAPTER 1

ANALGESIA AND PSYCHOTHERAPY

THE history of analgesia produced by psychological methods is extremely ancient.* However, it is not the intention here to consider the various magical procedures which have been used in primitive societies and which are found throughout the course of history. These practices were the appurtenances of the Priest or the Healer. Here we will trace the history of psychologically produced analgesia in the nineteenth century.†

It was toward the end of the eighteenth century that ANTOINE MESMER [362] became the first man to study the action of one individual upon another, an action which he considered due to a fluid, the 'magnetic fluid', which could flow between any two

---

*The Hebrews are supposed to have been acquainted with psychologically induced analgesia. The state in which Adam found himself during the creation of Eve has been given the word 'Tardemah' in the Hebrew text of the Bible. This word has been usually translated by the phrase 'deep sleep'. 'Tardemah' does not mean an ordinary sleep, it is sometimes translated by words such as lethargy, insensibility or trance (a 'trance-like sleep' in the dictionary of Jastrov). An American theologian, GLASNER [190] who studied the allusions to hypnosis in the Bible and the Talmud, has written concerning this sleep that 'It is tempting to surmise that the Biblical authors here reveal their familiarity with the use of hypnosis for anaesthesia'. He also describes the hypothesis of another author according to whom this word 'Tardemah' has been used several times in the Bible to describe a state which seems analogous to a hypnotic trance.

†GEORGE ROSEN [476], the editor of the *Journal of the History of Medicine*, has studied this period particularly in England. The paper published in this Journal was called 'Mesmerism and surgery; a strange chapter in the history of anaesthesia'. He shows that the proponents of mesmerism in surgery had drawn attention to the possibility of a surgery truly without pain. They thus prepared the way for the acceptance of ether and chloroform. A German author WALTER L. VON BRUNN [64], who has also studied this period, considers that this opinion of Rosen's is somewhat exaggerated. The French author EMILE ARON [21] in his *History of Anaesthesia* discusses hypnotic anaesthesia of the nineteenth century in his chapter entitled 'The beginning of the discovery'.

persons. His theory was incorrect, but in fact it allowed for an experimental study of phenomena which had previously been shrouded in mystery, and which were not accessible except to those who had been initiated. The action of animal magnetism showed itself chiefly by a convulsive crisis, which might have a salutory effect upon the patient. A pupil of Mesmer, the MARQUIS DE PUYSÉGUR [441] showed that this crisis was not always necessary and that the magnetizer could plunge the subject into a state of 'somnambulisme provoqué', in the course of which the subject remained in verbal contact with him.* This fluid theory was definitely refuted by BRAID [59] who introduced the term 'hypnotism'. Until then magnetic phenomena had been produced chiefly by hand passes, but largely owing to the work of Braid, and above all to that of LIÉBAULT [329], verbal suggestion became predominant. The foundations of modern psychotherapy were thus established.†

In the days of animal magnetism, the phenomenon of lack of sensibility in magnetized subjects was frequently observed. The first public demonstration of magnetic insensibility was made on 7 November 1820 on Husson's Unit at the Hôtel Dieu. The patient was Mlle Samson, a young woman of eighteen who was

---

*When de Puységur announced his discovery to Mesmer, the latter was not surprised. It is pretended that he had recognized it himself, but he dismissed any consideration of a psychological nature, wanting to keep his theory on a purely physiological level. For Mesmer the material action of a fluid analogous to electricity was the essential factor. He thus remained completely true to the spirit of mechanistic materialism of the eighteenth century. This mistrust of psychology was still in evidence at the end of the nineteenth century at the Saltpêtrière, where metallotherapy and transfer by magnets was still considered possible. A material agent must be found, rather than any psychological factor. When the importance of suggestion had been put forward by the Nancy group, Charcot's pupils, always mistrustful with regard to psychology, refused to study the work. Finally BABINSKI [28] announced the 'bankruptcy' of hypnosis.

†The ABBÉ FARIA [156] expressed himself strongly against the fluid theory of the Mesmeric School, considering that the essential feature of magnetism rested in the subject himself. He thus used verbal suggestion to put his subject to sleep. On the other hand, the technique of 'passes', detached from its fluid and magnetic background, is still employed today, paticularly by Russian authors (p.34).

magnetized by the Baron Du Potet. Récamier 'lifted her several times from the chair, pinched her, opened her eyes and yet she felt nothing'. Récamier continued his experiments and submitted two patients to the very painful application of a moxa. These patients were put to sleep by the magnetizer Robouam. The first experiment was made on 6 January 1821, a man called Starin was magnetized, then M. Récamier himself applied a moxa to the front and upper part of his right thigh; this produced an eschar of considerable size. The patient gave not the slightest sign of feeling, whether by groans, movements or changes in the pulse. On waking the pain was very intensely felt by the patient. The second experiment was made on 8 January, on a woman, Lise Leroy. Récamier placed a moxa on her epigastric region which 'produced an eschar of considerable size'. The reaction of the patient was identical to that seen in the first patient [163].

JULES CLOQUET was the first to undertake a surgical operation under magnetic anaesthesia on 12 April 1829. His communication was entitled 'The removal of a cancer of the breast whilst under magnetic sleep' and was given to the Académie Royale de Médecine on 16 April 1829 [96]. The patient, a woman of sixty-four and an asthmatic, was in poor general condition. Her doctor, Dr. Chapelain, put her into a somnambulistic state and in this state ordered her to 'undergo the operation without fear, in spite of the fact that during her waking moments she was filled with terror at the idea of an operation'. The operation lasted 12 minutes and, during it, the patient continued to converse quite calmly with the surgeon, giving not the slightest sign of any sensation. Cloquet's report unleashed the most passionate discussion, an occurrence which had been the usual course of events over the last fifty years whenever the subject of animal magnetism was brought up. In the course of this discussion Larrey, the former surgeon-in-chief of the Grande Armée, regretted that his fellow surgeon had allowed himself to be taken in by such trickeries. 'How can one tell,' he said, 'at what point interest or fanaticism can lead men to disguise their pains. The patient who was operated upon was nothing more than an accomplice of the somnambulizers'. Larrey himself reported amongst soldiers cases of loss of sensibility to pain in the course of major surgical interventions in the field. He attributed them to an effort of will. He thought this was also the case in the patient described by Cloquet, and that it was unnecessary to bring in any idea of a magnetic action. He quoted the case of Kléber's assassin who, in the middle of the most horrible tortures, did not stop singing. Although Larrey himself recognized the existence of a psychologically produced analgesia, he did not focus his discussion on the validity of this fact, but on the existence or absence of a magnetic action. In the same discussion Lisfranc quoted the case of a young woman in whom he was able to tie the carotid artery without the slightest sign of pain. Cloquet replied to these critics that he did not pretend to explain anything, that he only reported a fact and that 'truth as unbelievable as it may appear is none the less the truth and should always be reported'. He could only repeat the fact that this woman had been entirely impassive and shown the insensibility of a cataleptic or of a corpse during his operation. The Académie Royale de Médecine returned to this subject in a meeting on 24 January 1837. OUDET [406] described a case where dental intervention was undertaken under magnetic anaesthesia. This was, in effect, the case of a patient who was extremely sensitive to pain and on whom Oudet had carried out extraction under these conditions. An animated discussion followed in which Bouillaud, Roux and others took part. They all assured Oudet that he had been quite mistaken, as had Cloquet in 1829, remarking that there were no unequivocal signs allowing one to decide whether a patient was suffering or not.

Moreover the reasons for not expressing suffering could be manifold; Roux quoted the case of a patient who had a crop of vegetations on her genital organs. The patient presented herself masked to the doctor and did not utter one sound during the operation, which lasted for 15 minutes, for fear of betraying her incognito. Another time he amputated the breast of a young woman suffering from cancer. When he tried to get her to cry, believing that it was a good thing to express the feeling of pain, she replied, 'Oh sir, what are physical pains?' These writers quite well felt that in their patients the motivations for analgesia, or for a calm behaviour, were multiple and of a psychological order. This was not the problem; it was the question of magnetism.

Du Potet, the well-known Parisian magnetizer, arrived in

England in 1837 (where he was called the *prima donna* of the magnetic state) and there won over Elliotson, a very eminent doctor of the period, to the cause of magnetism. Elliotson encountered a very lively opposition on the part of his colleagues, and in 1838 the protector of Du Potet was forced to give up his official position in University College Hospital.* Elliotson devoted himself to the study and the propagation of animal magnetism from then on. In 1843 he founded a journal, the *Zoist*, which came to serve, until its last number in 1855, as the tribune for those who were interested in mesmerism in England. By means of the *Zoist* the mesmerizers were able to conduct their fight in the face of an active opposition. ELLIOTSON interested himself in magnetic analgesia and in 1843 published a collection of records of surgical operations carried out in England and other countries under magnetic influence [146]. From this date onwards the *Zoist* reported all surgical interventions in England and elsewhere which benefited from mesmeric anaesthesia.†

In India, ESDAILE was inspired by these reports, and in 1846 he reported seventy-five surgical operations under hypnotic anaesthesia [151]. In 1852 the number had risen to 315 [152]. Amongst others he removed 200 tumours of the scrotum, their weights varying between 10 and 103 lb. His technique was as follows: the magnetizers employed by Esdaile were young men, aged between fourteen and thirty, either Hindus or Mohammedans, the greater part of them surgical aides or pharmacists at the hospital at Hoogly, near Calcutta.‡ 'One mesmerizer was assigned to each patient. The room where they worked was kept dark, the patient lay on his back, naked to the waist, and with his legs uncovered. The magnetizer sitting at the head of the bed allowed his face to come almost into contact with that of the

*Elliotson had already incurred the hostility of his colleagues by his enthusiastic support of the stethoscope.

†At that time heated discussions took place in Great Britain on 'magnetic' analgesia and its authenticity. For instance the London *Medical Gazette* reported, on 18 December 1846 the use of ether in surgery in the United States under the title 'Animal Magnetism Superseded'.

‡Esdaile and Elliotson remained faithful to the 'fluid' theory. In spite of Braid's discoveries and the introduction of the word hypnotism (1843) the *Zoist* adhered to mesmerism and was antagonistic to the Manchester surgeon.

patient. His right hand was generally placed on the pit of the stomach and passes were made with one or both hands before the patient's face, chiefly concentrating on the eyes. The mesmerizer blew softly and frequently into the nose, between the lips and onto the eyes of the patient. The most profound silence was observed and the use of these procedures was continued for about two hours every day in all cases, even in one case for eight hours, and in another for six hours without interruption' [453].

In France at this time there were many surgical interventions under magnetic anaesthesia, for instance those of LOYSEL [335] of Cherbourg, RIBAUD and KIARO [see 331] and others. The discovery of ether, however, (1842–46), led to a diminished interest in magnetic anaesthesia. Elliotson and Esdaile had envisaged a still wider use of their method of anaesthesia; the advent of a pharmacodynamic anaesthesia destroyed all these hopes.

It was in the practical use of 'magnetic' analgesia that defeat occurred, not in its theoretical aspects. Paradoxically, the use of ether evoked arguments which confirmed the authenticity of hypnotic analgesia. In fact, HACK TUKE (1872), the grandson of William Tuke, the English *Pinel*, remarked 'that there was no delay in the recognition (during ether anaesthesia) that many phenomena like partial consciousness and cries caused by the apparent action of pain . . . were quite compatible with a perfect insensibility to pain and were not, as many people had considered, when mesmerism was in question, a proof of deceit' [543].

The important problem of the levels of integration of pain was raised: the subject's behaviour does not always reflect the degree of insensibility. This problem will be discussed again in the chapter relating to the various methods of psychological analgesia.

Braid's discovery was a turning point in the history of hypnosis; the technique changed once the hypnotic state could be obtained without passes, and purely by fixation on objects. Concerning analgesia, BRAID [59] wrote in 1843 that 'hypnotism lessens or entirely prevents pain in surgical operations'. He himself reported several operations, dental extractions, opening of abscesses, orthopaedic operations, etc., all of them carried out under hypnotic anaesthesia produced by his new technique. It was due to the work of Azam in Bordeaux that Braid's ideas were introduced into France. Azam spoke to Broca in 1859, but did not publish his work, according to Broca for the reason 'that in a subject as perilous as this, the excessive trickeries of the magnetizers rendered suspect to other men of science those who practised magnetism' BROCA, with FOLLIN, attempted in the latter's unit at l'Hôpital Necker, an operation under hypnotic anaesthesia produced by Braid's technique. They described their experience in the Académie des Sciences [62] on 5 December 1859 and two days later to the Société de Chirurgie [63]. The patient had 'a large and extremely painful abscess at the margin of the anus. M. Follin opened up the abscess which gave issue to an enormous quantity of fetid pus. A slight cry which lasted less than a second was the only sign which the patient gave of all these occurrences'. There was, on waking, a complete amnesia. Broca seemed to have feared certain accidents which might be caused by chemical analgesia. 'As things are,' he wrote, 'the surgeon does not want to be the author of the latest observation on death from chloroform, and so all the harmless methods which may succeed even on one occasion deserve to be studied'. Nevertheless he had no illusions with regard to the general use of hypnotic procedures in surgery. However extraordinary they appear, 'they deserve the attention of physiologists even though they are not constant enough to act as a foundation for a regular method of surgical anaesthesia. The study of hypnotism is one which will, without doubt, bring an increase in knowledge to our understanding of physiology'. Theories of suggestion were still not generally recognized. Broca suspected the identity of the condition produced by the magnetizer's procedure and that obtained by Braid's methods. 'In his important report on elephantiasis of the scrotum M. Larrey[*] has spoken to us of the numerous operations practised by a surgeon in Calcutta under mesmeric anaesthesia. When I remember that the face of the mesmerist remains immobile and balanced on top of the patient's face for quite a long time I am tempted to attribute this solely to the same cause, to bring it into line in consequence of

---

[*]He spoke of Hippolyte Larrey, son of Napoleon's surgeon, who contrary to his father, seems to have recognized the reality of hypnotic anaesthesia.

this with the procedure initiated by M. Braid'.* Broca was far from 'believing that this latter procedure was the only one which brought forth the phenomena of catalepsy, hyperaesthesia and anaesthesia, which really constitute the hypnotic state'. He recognized without naming it the phenomenon of group suggestion when speaking of imitation and of contagion, both of which can produce analogous results.

The Nuns of Loudun, the Ecstatics of the Cévennes and the baquet of Mesmer† are 'further examples of the facility with which the functions of the central nervous system can be disturbed in certain subjects'. Broca expressed ideas which were to be confirmed later by modern dynamic psychology on the overlapping of normal and pathological states: 'I think that this aptitude has shown how under the influence of causes apparently slight, a severe disturbance of the functions of the central nervous system can be produced, and that it occurs in a more or less developed way in the majority, and perhaps even in all individuals'. Hypnosis can thus be produced in everyone, without it necessarily being a pathological state. This problem will be discussed later when describing the relationships between hysteria and hypnosis, which were so hotly debated between the Nancy School and that of Charcot. In the discussion which followed Broca's communication the objection was made that in this case surgery was confined really to a simple incision, yet nevertheless a cry was uttered by the patient. Broca protested that this interpretation was wrong. He spoke of operating on a large, very painful abscess in the anal region. The cries of the patient proved nothing. Patients who were submitted to chloroform anaesthesia cried and became agitated when they were operated upon. 'The important thing is that at the moment of awakening they have no memory of what has happened and often doubt whether the operation has actually taken place'.

Meanwhile in 1859, Guérineau [211] of Poitiers published a

*Broca also reported that according to Braid, the sculptors of ancient time had recourse to some procedure which was analogous to hypnotism, so as to render their models cataleptic and thus assure the immobility of their poses.

†A modern replica of these phenomena can be seen today particularly in young people who practise or listen to the new 'rock and roll' rhythm.

case of amputation of the thigh carried out under hypnotic anaesthesia.

As early as 1860 LIÉBAULT carried out tooth extractions and minor operations under hypnotic analgesia; he introduced a new approach which was to have important theoretical and practical consequences. He demonstrated the possibility of inducing analgesia through post-hypnotic suggestion, later called *suggestion à terme*. 'It was possible', he wrote, 'to extract teeth or perform other minor operations, after awakening'. In 1882–1883 he gave post-hypnotic suggestions of analgesia to nineteen subjects who later went to the dentist and underwent a painless or nearly painless extraction. Liebault considered that the interval between hypnosis and the operation should be short, but it could be longer, especially in good subjects.

In 1887 LIÉBAULT again emphasized the method of post-hypnotic analgesia which he used with LIÉGEOIS for tooth extractions. The suggestion was made at various depths of trance and the subjects 'failed to feel any pain when these minor operations were performed, even a long time after waking'. [330].

In the great period of hypnosis from 1880–1895, experiments on hypnotic analgesia were further pursued. In France, PITRES [420], MABILLIE and RAMADIER [342], (these three authors produced analgesia by post-hypnotic suggestion, at this period described as 'suggestions à terme'—the operation was undertaken in a waking state), BERNHEIM [42] (analgesia by suggestion in the waking state), FORT [168], MESNET [364], and LIÉGEOIS [331] (dental extraction by post-hypnotic suggestion). In Switzerland, FOREL [167], in the U.S.A. WOOD [579], in Sweden VELANDER [550], in Cuba AUARD MARTINEZ DIAZ [79] reported similar cases. Other observations of hypnotic anaesthesia in surgery present an interest purely experimental and were published sporadically. The two latest have been published in England by MASON [350] and in the U.S.A. by KROGER and DE LEE [288]. Hypnosis is now used by certain anaesthetists as an occasional adjuvant for pharmacological anaesthesia, and in particular to obtain a pre-operative sedation as well as a post-operative analgesia [312, 313, 407, 446, 587]. At the close of this brief survey, it must be emphasized that the communications of Cloquet, Oudet and Broca, and the ensuing discussions had already posed the problem of the experimental aspect of pain, and of the value of psychological analgesia.

Now what relationship do these reports have to painless childbirth? From the psychophysiological point of view there is little difference qualitatively between the production of an experimental analgesia by hypnotic means and the production of analgesia by other psychological means. There is only a difference of degree. In experimental hypnotic anaesthesia or in hysterical anaesthesia, phenomena are seen as through a magnifying glass. In the case of hysteria the pathological process creates nothing new, it either exaggerates or diminishes a state which is already in existence.* We will see later that the clinical experiences of hypnotic analgesia have provided Russian authors with a foundation for their new method of psychoprophylaxis. The first deliveries under hypnotic sleep were performed toward the middle of the nineteenth century. The first attempts to produce obstetrical analgesia in subjects in a somnambulistic state revealed psychophysiological problems which are today still being studied in the modern psychosomatic methods of preparation for childbirth.

*This is a much debated problem. Essentially, we will not consider the action of the hypnosuggestive and the educative methods as identical. In the educative methods, if suggestion plays a part in the production of the analgesia, other factors of an educational nature, working at different levels, can equally well lessen the pain of childbirth. This problem will be discussed later.

CHAPTER 2

THE FIRST OBSTETRICAL ANALGESIAS PRODUCED BY HYPNOSUGGESTIVE TECHNIQUES

OBSTETRICAL analgesia produced by a magnetic influence was first mentioned by FOISSAC [163] in his 'explanatory notes' which accompanied the celebrated report of Husson* (1831) on the magnetic experiments made before the Commission of the Royal Academy of Medicine. 'A small number of observations gives us ground for hoping that it will be possible to modify, by these means, the sometimes intolerable pains of labour'.

Du Potet reported in the *Journal du Magnétisme*, the experience of Dr. Cutter of Nashua (New Hampshire) in the U.S.A. using magnetic treatment in a woman in labour.

'In June 1837 I was called to see Mrs. Fern, who had been in labour for 48 hours. The rhythm of the pains was irregular, and she had not slept for three nights. At her request and in the presence of Mesdames Lawrence and Waston, I magnetized her. She fell into a magnetic sleep in less than a minute. I ought to say that I had never previously seen this patient. The sleep was very peaceful and she slept about three hours. On waking she was much relieved. To my own surprise and the astonishment of the two ladies, we observed this interesting fact and phenomenon, to wit: the special and regular contractions of the uterus which accompany labour continued with perfect regularity' [108].

DU POTET published in this same journal in 1852, an extract from the *Zoist* (No. 38), the English periodical devoted to magnetism, containing a letter addressed to Dr. Elliotson by Dr. S. D. Saunders, of Back Hall, Bristol. His wife, magnetized

---

*It is of some interest that the Commission set up by the British Medical Association to report on the 'Medical uses of hypnosis', published in 1955, commented at length on the Husson report. It considered that his conclusions showed 'a remarkable foresight, they are, in large part, still applicable today' [466, 81].

by himself, had gone through her childbirth in a magnetic sleep, experiencing no pain whatever [488].

CH. LAFONTAINE* of Geneva, the well-known magnetizer, reported a delivery carried out in 1843 in a somnambulistic state in his book *L'Art de Magnétiser ou le Magnétisme Animal* [291]. He intervened 15 minutes before delivery and put the woman in a somnambulistic state. Analgesia was not obtained, but on waking up, the woman had no recollection of the delivery. In the same book Lafontaine quotes a letter from Dr. Fauconnet, dated 1860, reporting a case of obstetrical analgesia, induced by Lafontaine. The patient, aged twenty-five, was a hysteric. The intervention began at the beginning of the period of dilatation. 'Madame M. . . . continued to feel the uterine contractions which she announced every time she felt them, but without feeling the slightest sensation of pain: her face remained calm and smiling and she continued the conversation whilst the contractions were going on'.

LIÉBAULT [329] in his book *Du Sommeil et des Etats Analogues* (1866) writes of his own experiences in the chapter entitled 'L'insensibilité des dormeurs utilisée pour favoriser des opérations chirurgicales ou un travail physiologique douloureux'. He had four cases of childbirth—the first was delivered 'in a deep sleep, in which the woman remained for 22 hours; she experienced all the contractions, in spite of my suggestions to the contrary. She maintained, however, that she did not feel them as acutely as in her previous labours. On waking up, she recalled her last three pains, and the groans she had uttered at the same time'. The same findings were present in another woman, a somnambulist put to sleep in quite an advanced stage of labour. The third woman was put into a trance towards the end of her labour, but was woken by the contractions. The fourth 'a professional somnambulist', was plunged into a deep sleep but had to be awakened after half an hour because she did not experience much relief.

Liébault, not having obtained a complete loss of sensation, considered that his results were not encouraging. Nevertheless he writes 'It is quite clear that they maintained that they had

---

*It was after seeing a public demonstration by Lafontaine in Manchester that Braid first became interested in animal magnetism.

suffered less than usual, and that, of the four, three did not wake up in spite of the pains'. He concluded that 'this slight success is not sufficient for us to hold the belief that painless childbirth does not occur in sleep'.

In 1882 he prepared a woman for several weeks with hypnosuggestions; he failed to obtain a completely painless childbirth, but the duration of her labour (in previous deliveries lasting 48 hours) was 'reduced to 13 hours of suffering'. This was her sixth childbirth; she had always suffered from uterine inertia and profuse bleeding. LIÉBAULT thought that he had influenced the physiology of childbirth, more than the pain itself [327] and he attributed this influence to suggestion. 'If it could be objected', he stated, 'that, exceptionally, the course of events might have been different if the properties of sleep had not been resorted to, it must be confessed that it is very likely that the result was due to the hypnotic use of suggestion'.

In 1887 he reported two new cases of obstetrical analgesia through suggestion: 'The patients were both put into a state of somnambulism, hardly suffered and had no memory, only one of them recalling some contractions at the end of delivery.' [328]. LIÉBAULT also used suggestion in the 'treatment of the disorders complicating pregnancy, delivery and the post-delivery period'. and mentioned lumbar pains, vomiting and other disorders related to pregnancy. He laid particular emphasis on a case treated in 1875: a woman expecting her sixth child had complained, following each very painful delivery, of extremely violent uterine pain, worse than the strongest contractions felt during childbirth itself. Following the use of his suggestive treatment, these pains failed to recur. In reply to those who might argue that this result was due to the action of suggestion he wrote, 'It is strange that the above symptoms, identical at each childbirth, and occurring five times in succession, had stopped at the sixth childbirth'. [328].

The first observations of Lafontaine and Liébault present a group of problems which have continued to preoccupy those physiologists and psychologists who strive to understand the mechanisms of psychotherapeutically produced analgesia. A mechanism resulting from a psychological or verbal action of one individual on another produces a relief of pain. This relief is, however, variable. For instance, it is possible to feel the uterine contractions without the least sensation of pain; the pain can be diminished; in spite of the pain, the behaviour remains calm, the patient can forget.

Liébault discusses the mechanism behind this analgesia and writes 'From the moment when, chiefly in somnambulism, the attention is forced back toward the brain and is firmly fixed on a memory, there is nothing surprising in the ensuing loss of feeling. Similar mental states are met with in which most remarkable sensory changes are found; for instance in psychotics, in soldiers during the heat of battle, and even in some lively personalities, as well as in those who from pure *sang froid* possess the ability to render themselves insensible by shifting their attention as did Campanella* to ideas other than that of the pain, or in maintaining a denial of their trouble'.

Liébault describes in simple language the process of analgesia: attention can be focused on ideas other than those concerning pain. This hypothesis is still valid. The Pavlovians have formulated this in their concepts of excitation and inhibition; modern neurophysiologists are now applying experimental techniques to the study of attention (p. 188).

The work of Liébault, appearing in 1866, attracted little attention in the world of medicine. It was only 20 years later, thanks to the labours of BERNHEIM [42], BEAUNSIS [34] and LIÉGEOIS [331] that his ideas began to be reckoned with. The great period of hypnosis began about 1878 and was marked by the battle between the Nancy School and the Saltpêtrière group. For CHARCOT [77] hypnosis was nothing but an artificial hysteria, a pathological state, with its three phases, catalepsy, lethargy and somnambulism. The Nancy School was of the opposite view: hypnosis was not a pathological state, it could be produced amongst perfectly normal subjects.

---

*Campanella, the author of the *Cité du Soleil*, was an Italian philosopher usually considered to have been a pioneer of socialism. He spent 27 years in prison.

CHAPTER 3

HYPNOSUGGESTIVE METHODS IN OBSTETRICS AT THE END OF THE 19th CENTURY

TOWARDS the end of the nineteenth century, the research workers who were investigating the use of hypnosis in obstetrical analgesia had been, for the most part, influenced by the school of Charcot. Their experiments were therefore limited to hysterical subjects and the number of cases they studied was very small. Their observations, however, were extremely detailed and all the women's reactions were noted down with great precision. The artificial division of hypnosis into different phases, very strictly defined, nevertheless brought in useless complications.

In 1885 Pritzl, of Vienna, described the use of hypnosis in suppressing the pain of childbirth.

In 1888 AUVARD and SECHEYRON [25] published a review in which they discussed those cases which had been studied by AUVARD and VARNIER [26], VARNIER and SECHEYRON [549], DUMONTPALLIER [137], MESNET [363] and THOMAS [528], and also reported the observations of PRITZL [436] of Vienna and of FÉRÉ and BUDIN [158] and of PORAK [431].

A certain number of interesting points can be found in this paper relating to problems which were to be discussed years later.

1. TECHNIQUE

The hypnotic state was obtained either by tactile stimulation (placing the hands on the shoulders, pressure on the eyeballs) or by visual means (fixation on a bright light or on a metal ball), or by verbal suggestion. Luys used an arrangement of mirrors in his technique.

The analgesia was obtained either spontaneously or following definite suggestion. Indirect suggestions were also brought in as by abdominal and lumbar massage, or by breathing through a pad soaked in perfumed liquid; the procedure was either extemporary or preceded by a more or less lengthy training. It was sometimes found that a woman was hypnotizable during her period of preparation, but not at the moment of childbirth.*

2. RESULTS

The objective criteria used for assessing diminution of pain sensation is a cardinal problem. AUVARD and SECHEYRON [25] consider 'that it would be very difficult to dissimulate the pains, to appear to sleep in such a painful situation. The pains of childbirth can hardly be misleading as a criterion'. They doubt the reliability of reports of patients themselves, owing to the retrospective amnesia. The degree of insensibility varies, sometimes being complete and accompanied by amnesia for the labour, sometimes the contractions are felt, but the woman does not suffer; yet again the patient groans, suffers, but remains under control. The labour may also be painful and disturbing, but followed by amnesia.

---

*The analgesiant procedure used by the American dentist BONWILL must be reported [54]. From 1875 on, he let the patient practise rapid breathing (up to a hundred respiratory movements per minute) and thus obtained a sufficient analgesia for tooth extractions and for minor operations of short duration. Bonwill reported that this method was also used by Hewson [316] to suppress the pain of childbirth, and at the same time Lee published a paper in which he wrote favourably of anaesthesia with compulsory, rapid breathing. BLANCHARD, who reported these facts in France, *Progrés Médical* [45] related that a dentist of Monaco performed fifteen extractions with this method.

To explain the mechanism of the analgesia, Bonwill suggested that attention was diverted on to the breathing, and that hypercapnia was also important, the latter possibly inducing a cloudy state of consciousness with insensibility to pain.

Lee mentions partial hypnotism through fixation of attention. Recounting Bonwill's experiments in *L'Encephale*, PETIT considers that Wayman's views were identical [412]. Thus, 'the same kind of hypnotism would be involved as that obtained by gazing steadily at a bright object placed near the eyes'.

SARGENT and FRAZER [487] describe a procedure of hypnotism through hyperventilation leading to a lowering of the level of consciousness with increased suggestibility due to blood alkalosis. STOKVIS regards this procedure as hypnotization by means of auto-toxic stimuli [512].

Certain writers consider that the frequency and length of the contractions can be modified. DUMONTPALLIER [137] states that under hypnosis the contractions are longer and less frequent, although these findings have not been confirmed by others. Auvard and Secheyron obtained complete analgesia in four of thirteen women, partial in four, and failure in the remaining five. They counsel caution with regard to hypnosis largely as they dealt with neurotic, sometimes psychotic women. Also, for medico-legal reasons they only very exceptionally advise hypnosis.

JULES CHAIGNEAU [75] reached similar conclusions in his thesis. This work shows the influence of the Saltpêtrière group, and its limitation of hypnosis to hysterics: 'Hypnotism ought never to be used in women who do not present unequivocal symptoms of hysteria'. FRAIPONT and DELBŒUF [169] attempted to bring back, by suggestion, contractions which were becoming weaker and to establish a rhythm, every four minutes. Moreover, the suggestion was made that lactation should occur by the end of the third day of childbirth.*

FANTON [155] of Marseilles claims to have regulated the frequency and length of the contractions. DUMONTPALLIER [138] was the first to practise autohypnosis with one of his patients. He also obtained analgesia by suggestion in a waking state. LE MENANT DE CHESNAIS [319] determined by suggestion the precise hour of delivery.

Other French writers describing the use of hypnosis in obstetrical analgesia in the period 1880–1900 include DE GRANDCHAMPS [198], LUYS [338, 339], BLANCHE EDWARDS [144], JOURNÉE [257], VOISIN [565], LUGEOL [336]. WETTERSTRAND [575] in Sweden, KINGSBURY [265] in England, SALLIS [486], SCHRENK-NOTZING [496], TATZEL [522] in Germany, DOBROVOLSKY [129], BOTKINE [55], MATVEEV [351], WIAZEMSKY [576] in Russia, DE

*LIÉBAULT had already reported an increase in milk secretion [329] through suggestion. FREUD [174] himself obtained lactation by suggestion under hypnosis in one of his patients who could not feed her baby and who was very disturbed by this. GROSSMANN [206] of Koenitz, re-established lactation which had ceased. LUYS [340] experimentally produced a mammary secretion in a woman who was not lactating. Some Russian writers still employ this technique even today. LICHTSCHEIN [328] also regulated the secretion of the mammary gland by hyposuggestion.

JONG [254] in Holland, and RAMON CAJAL [448] in Spain all used hypnotically produced obstetrical analgesia.

In the United States, LICHTSCHEIN [328] tried hypnotic analgesia in forty-eight parturient women; nine could not be hypnotized. Some of them delivered under hypnosis; others woke up during strong contractions, but the post-hypnotic effect of suggestion nevertheless relieved pain.

After the death of Charcot, the discredit into which hypnosis fell in France led research workers to turn to methods of suggestion in a waking state, without having recourse to hypnosis. JOIRE [253] of Lille developed a method which he described as follows: 'The technique is simple. One hand is placed on the subject's eyes, whose eyelids close spontaneously under this light touch. The other hand is placed on the abdomen, and at the same time verbal suggestions are made, softly, slowly, persuasively without in any way giving the impression of implanting in the patient's mind a wish or an idea which insinuates itself softly, which she accepts, and which she makes effective without questioning that she is accepting suggestion'.*

*The replacement of hypnosis by 'laying on of hands' was used by Freud. He had seen Bernheim recover a post-hypnotic amnesia by this method, and in his turn, on giving up hypnosis, and before introducing his psychoanalytic technique, Freud found it useful. He wrote 'This certainly ought to be more disturbing than to put someone into a hypnotic state' [177]. The German worker FLOEL [161] used this technique in obstetrics, and contrary to Freud, found it easier than hypnosis.

CHAPTER 4

EVOLUTION OF THE CONCEPTION OF HYPNOSIS

THE foundations of modern psychotherapy were created in the great period of hypnosis 1880–1890. Charcot stressed the importance of the psychological component in the genesis of hysterical disorders.*

A psychological disorder can produce somatic symptoms; hysterical anaesthesia is thus related to a psychological occurrence; anaesthesia can be produced by psychological action. Charcot considered that hypnosis was an artificial hysteria; Bernheim on

*'It must be recognized that hysteria is a psychological illness,' wrote the illustrious Master of the Saltpêtrière (*Ed. Polycopiée*, 1887, Vol. 1, p. 207, cited by Janet in 'J.-M. Charcot, son oeuvre psychologique', *Revue Philosophique de la France et de l'étranger*, 1895, Vol. 39, pp. 567–604. This saying of Charcot cannot be found in the printed edition of the *Lecons du Mardi*, Vol. 1 published in 1892.) FREUD [175] states that Charcot was the first to give an explanation of the mechanism of hysteria. Charcot, Freud writes, had the idea of reproducing the paralyses which occur in post traumatic hysterical states in patients who had been put into a somnambulistic state. Charcot succeeded in demonstrating that 'these paralyses are the result of ideas which have dominated the patient's brain, which was already in a special state'. This 'beautiful piece of clinical research' helped Janet and Breuer to build up their theory of neurosis, so Freud believes [175].

GUILLAIN [212] in a recent study of Charcot mentions Pierre Marie's opinion that the work on hypnotism was 'a slight lapse' on the part of Charcot, but Guillain finds extenuating circumstances for this 'slight lapse'. In his opinion, even if Charcot's works on hypnotism can be criticized on several grounds, they have not been useless and without value; they are still of importance therapeutically and from the medicolegal point of view. Moreover these researches have influenced later work on psychoanalysis. Before mentioning Freud's statement (which we have just quoted), Guillain also mentions Janet's opinion: 'Charcot's lectures on the traumatic neuroses and my own studies have been the starting point for a whole most remarkable study on the interpretation of neuroses and their treatment. I am speaking of the studies on psychoanalysis carried out by Professor Freud at Vienna and by his numerous pupils' [247].

the other hand maintained that hypnosis was not hysteria, unless everybody had a little of the hysterical in his make-up. In fact, modern dynamic psychology has established the view that each type of pathological personality is only an accentuation of what is normal. In order to understand normal psychology it is possible to start from the pathological.*

DELAY formulates this viewpoint when he writes: 'the pathological method allows us to understand better than anything else the architecture of mental functions. The illness is, as it were, a vivisection which presents stage by stage, level by level, an atlas of mental anatomy' [118].

FERENCZI [159] a pupil of Freud, using the discoveries of his master on the transference situation, brought new perspectives to bear which in some way ought to have bridged the gap between the ideas of Charcot and those of Bernheim. He shared Bernheim's views on suggestibility but believed that the idea so firmly fixed in scientific circles that Charcot's conception of hypnosis was absurd ought to be revised. Hypnosis can in fact be related to an artificial hysteria inasmuch as the same psychological mechanisms are found in the production of either one or the other. The hysterical symptoms as well as the hypnotic phenomena are produced as a result of emotions felt by the subject in the first case in regard to a significant person in his past and in the second case to the hypnotist himself. Ferenczi quotes Jung, for whom 'well balanced individuals struggle with the same complexes which make neurotic individuals ill'. He notes that the hypnotist can

---

*CHARCOT wrote: 'According to this well-established law that pathological manifestations do not embody in themselves any new elements, they are only deviations, modifications, more or less profound, of physiological conditions; it therefore follows that regarded in this way morbid phenomena are full of significance from the physiological point of view and that the illness often reveals secrets of the normal state. Hypnotism is, as it were, a means of experimentation in the regular functioning of the organism and the spontaneous disorders which arise from the illness. The hypnotic state is nothing else than an artificial or experimental nervous state whose many manifestations either appear or vanish according to the needs of the research and at the will of the observer. Considered in this sort of way, hypnotism becomes a precious source to be exploited just as much by the physiologist and the psychologist as by the doctor' [78].

produce neither more nor less than the neurosis produces spontaneously. On the other hand Pavlovian teaching also considers that the physiological mechanism of hypnosis is the same as that of hysteria, to wit, the processes of inhibition and phasic states.

The researches of the Pavlovian School on sleep have determined the theory with regard to hypnosis. It is the cortex which plays the determining role in the production of sleep. There are two processes at work with regard to cerebral activity, excitation and inhibition, and it is these two processes which, with the help of temporary connections (conditioned reflexes) adapt the organism to the external world. When the excitatory process exhausts the neurone, inhibition sets in, in order to protect it. Sleep is based on inhibition. Hypnosis is an intermediate state between waking and sleeping; it is partial sleep, a partial inhibition, just as much from the topographical point of view as from the point of view of intensity. In the cortex there are 'waking points' which in man allow for the development of the relationship between the hypnotist and his subject. Hypnosis comprises three phases which are termed hypnoid phases. They are the phase of equalization, the paradoxical phase and the ultraparadoxical phase. In the phase of equalization every conditioned excitant, whether strong or weak, acts in a similar way; in the paradoxical phase a strong excitant provokes a weak or null reaction, and vice versa, the weak excitant provokes a strong reaction. In the ultraparadoxical phase, a reaction can be obtained by a negative stimulus, that is to say by a stimulus to which the cerebral neurones would not react in a waking state. In this way the phenomena of hypnotic anaesthesia which can be obtained in the paradoxical phase can be understood. Pavlov called it the phase of suggestion, and it is simple in this phase to suppress harmful reflexes and to implant other positive ones. In his interpretation of Pavlov's ideas, PLATONOV [558] explains that the phasic states are fleeting under physiological conditions, but that they can persist for weeks or months in pathological conditions. These hypnoid phases can thus be considered on the one hand as the physiological substrate of neuroses or of psychoses, but on the other hand 'they present a normal form of the physiological battle against the morbid agent (hypnosis)'. It can be seen that these explanatory hypotheses, psychological and physiological, query the view that hypnotic phenomena are essentially pathological in nature.

The dispute between the Nancy School and the Saltpêtrière killed hypnosis in France, where it hardly survived the death of Charcot (1893). It is always difficult to bring about a synthesis between the physiological and the psychological, and this is the stumbling block in researches on hypnosis. After the collapse of the three stage theory of 'Grand Hypnotisme' developed by Charcot, and in the absence of precise signs, there was a reaction on the part of his pupils, for whom psychological theories were too vague. Their desire for a clear physiological understanding did not however come to fruition. Hypnotism being applied either wrongly or in a distorted way, after the original exaggerated enthusiasm a very marked scepticism arose. The reality of hypnotic phenomena even came to be disputed and Babinski, about 1910, declared that it was nothing less than a semi-simulation. Hypnosis was completely abandoned in France and JANET alone maintained his interest in it. He believed that it was going through 'a temporary eclipse' [24]; the result of a 'temporary accident in the history of somnambulism and in the history of psychotherapy' [248]. In other countries the decline of hypnosis was less acute, Bernheim's ideas lived on and hypnosis began to be applied to normal subjects. The inadequacy of hypnosis gave birth to psychoanalysis, the latter giving a new psychological explanation to the former. Then considering that its therapeutic effects were too superficial, psychoanalysis also gave it up. After the first world war there was a renewal of interest in hypnosis, for hypnotherapy had proved itself of value in the treatment of war neuroses. Studies on hypnosis increased, particularly in Central Europe, in the Soviet Union and in the United States. Hypnosis was no longer considered as a pathological phenomenon, and as a result hypnosuggestive analgesia has come to be applied to normal subjects.

CHAPTER 5

HYPNOSUGGESTIVE METHODS IN GERMANY AND AUSTRIA AFTER THE FIRST WORLD WAR

A NEW wave of interest in hypnosis was manifest in Germany and Austria after the First World War. There were three reasons for this: (1) the successful use of hypnotic techniques in military psychiatry during the war, and (2) the changing concept of hypnosis which was now, in general, considered to be a normal phenomenon (3). The progress realized in the explanation of physical disorders by psychogenesis, thanks to the studies of Freud, Adler, Stekel and others.*

Psychotherapy was applied in gynaecology, and hypnosis, as one form of psychotherapy, came into use. Hypnotherapy was employed not only in the treatment of functional gynaecological and obstetrical disorders but also to induce analgesia in minor operations (Raefler, Raefler and Schultze Rhonhof, etc. . .). And, lastly, hypnotic analgesia was carried out for childbirth itself at the time when a reaction was occurring against the ill effects of 'twilight sleep' produced by the opiates (morphine–scopolamine mixtures). The introduction of twilight sleep had produced a brisk controversy in medical circles, kindled in the press and by public opinion. Some journals went so far as to propose obligatory analgesia for all women in childbirth. Medical men violently opposed this view, citing the dangers to the mother and to the child. Some doctors even refused to consider that there was a true analgesia, having produced only a state of restlessness in their patients, and only seeing an amnesia as the result of the treatment. Moral reasons were also adduced against the method: the woman was deprived of experiencing an event of the greatest importance to her emotional life (NASSAUER [378]).

---
*Some twenty years later this trend will be called 'Psychosomatic Medicine'. The important book of O. Schwarz was published in 1925, and could be qualified 'Psychosomatic': *Psychogenese und Psychotherapie Körperlicher Symptome.*

But ZWEIFEL was opposed to the idea that painful delivery could be considered a major event in a woman's life. A partisan of 'Dämmerschlaf', he considered that pain which was not remembered had not, so to say, existed. Complete analgesia could be induced, according to this author, only if it is accompanied by amnesia. Without amnesia, only a decrease in pain was obtained [586].

During this brief period from 1920 to 1923, numerous theoretical and practical problems of psychologically induced analgesia were debated by obstetricians and psychiatrists. The discussions to which they gave rise have remained unsolved to the present day. But the techniques employed at that time were, in effect, very close to those in use today. They consisted of the use of hypnosis either during delivery, or in the phase of preparation for childbirth, or were a combination of hypnosis and medication, or lastly of suggestion in a waking state.

BONNE [52], an army doctor, used hypnosis during the war. By hypnotizing the patient before giving a narcotic, he was able to reduce the quantity of the anaesthetic agent, and to suppress the state of excitement at the beginning of anaesthesia (generally, at this time, chloroform). GUECKEL [207], of Nuremberg, had used a psychotherapeutic approach to anaesthesia since 1915 and had potentiated the action of chloroform and ether by the use of suggestion at the time when the patient was put to sleep. The stage of excitement was suppressed and he was able to reduce the toxic effects associated with surgical anaesthesia by as much as a third or even a half. FRIEDLANDER [180] also elaborated a technique of hypnonarcosis, based on the same principles as in the methods used by Bonne and Gueckel.

A number of publications concerned the use of hypnosis and suggestion in obstetrics; VON OETTINGEN [405], HEBERER [224], KIRSTEIN [267], HALLAUER [217], FLOEL [161], FALK [153], FRIGYESI and MANSFELD [182] of Budapest, KROENIG and SCHOENHOLZ [282]. The most important were those of SCHULTZE-RHONHOF [499, 500] and of KOGERER [275, 276]. Lively controversies took place on the techniques advocated by the different writers. These were aired at the 17th Congress of the German Society of Gynaecology, held at Innsbruck in June 1922 [101]. The use of hypnosis in obstetrics was first begun by VON OETTINGEN at Heidelberg. His first publication [405] reported 16 patients, in 14 of whom he had had good results. The women were delivered under hypnosis; amnesia was complete in six women, partial in eight. During the contractions the women moaned only slightly. Drugs were used in order to reinforce the analgesia. At the same clinic in Heidelberg, SCHULTZE-RHONHOF [499, 500] further developed von Oettingen's technique. He omitted drugs, and dispensed with the amnesia. At least four sessions were given during pregnancy to a preparation of the patients for childbirth. They were group sessions, and no importance was attached to their spacing nor to the date of the first and last sessions. He considered that the group method saved time, and also enhanced the quality of the suggestions which were made. Before taking part in their own preparation, the women 'sat-in' at another group meeting. Hypnosis was preceded by an introduction, during the course of which the doctor explained to the patients just what hypnosis was, in such a way as to relieve them of any erroneous ideas that they might have on the subject. They were told that hypnosis resembled normal sleep, with the difference, however, that the patient remained in touch with her doctor throughout. The first treatment was aimed at producing a light trance, with suggestions of heaviness and fatigue. In the ensuing sessions the trance was deepened, with suggestions being made regarding anaesthesia, amnesia and posthypnotic suggestions. One of these latter was that the woman should come to the labour room when contractions were felt at intervals of 10–15 minutes. The patient was then hypnotized in the interval between the contractions.

After the birth and the evacuation of the placenta, the patient's eyes were opened, and her child shown to her. By appropriate suggestions the amnesia and analgesia were made to disappear, and the patient was then awakened. During the course of labour, some women uttered a slight groan, others showed some agitation, all of them maintained, however, on waking up, that they had not suffered at all.

Schultze-Rhonhof asked himself whether these manifestations were the result of a true analgesia, or of an amnesia, and after a series of experiments, concluded that taking the whole process of childbirth into account 'suggestion produces not only an

amnesia, but an effective diminution of pain, and in certain cases, its complete suppression. But this last is unusual. In the majority of cases, the complete analgesia which is claimed on waking is the result of the amnesia.' He added that even if suggestion only produced amnesia, it was of value with regard to future experiences of childbirth [499]. Schultze-Rhonhof also carried out obstetrical manoeuvres and operations under hypnotic analgesia. Out of 79 patients, 80 per cent gave a good result; 70 women declared that they had either amnesia or analgesia. The objection was made that the use of this method demanded the presence of a doctor trained in the technique. Accordingly all the doctors in the clinic were made familiar with hypnotic techniques. Later, autohypnosis by posthypnotic suggestion was tried, coming into effect as soon as the women got into bed in the labour room.*
As to the depth of hypnosis, a very high percentage of deep trance states was obtained.

HEBERER [224] of Dresden published 50 cases of women delivered under hypnosis with good results as to analgesia; in order to let the woman take part in the birth he woke her during the expulsion of the shoulders. He believed that the questioning of the women ought never to be done by her therapist, because the answers could be given wrongly out of a desire to please. In his published figures there were seven with a contracted pelvis, two breeches and one twin birth. He was able to carry out five episiotomies, and two forceps deliveries under hypnosis.

The Viennese psychiatrist KOGERER [275, 276] described a technique using hypnosis alone in preparation for labour, and in which analgesia was obtained by means of posthypnotic suggestion, the woman delivering herself in the waking state. He had been struck by a detail recorded by von Oettingen. Certain women arrived late at the labour ward, after the rupture of the membranes, because they had felt no contractions. One of these had delivered herself in a waking state; without feeling pain. Von Oettingen had paid little attention to this, and had not even recorded it as a success. Kogerer, on the contrary, saw in this a solution to

---

*This procedure had been already used by DUMONTPALLIER [138] in 1891.

the problem. It was possible to avoid hypnosis at the moment of birth and thereby not deprive the mother of participating in it.

Kogerer began to prepare the woman two or three weeks before the expected date of delivery. The number of sessions varied, and he had observed painless childbirth after three or four sessions. He attempted to divest hypnosis of all its spectacular and magical aspects. He explained to the women that hypnosis was a normal happening, an incomplete sleep in the course of which 'one dreams and one is aware that one dreams', whilst contact was still maintained with the surrounding world. He used ocular fixation and verbal suggestions; after producing the first hypnotic manifestations (heaviness and closing of the lids, and tiredness) he suggested a limb paralysis, in order to show the woman that suggestion could produce physical effects. He repeatedly told her that she could wake up if she wanted to do so. He then suggested an analgesia of the skin on the dorsum of the hand, then of the abdomen. The woman was delivered in the waking state. After the birth, in a last session, he removed the suggestions he had made previously. Kogerer considered that pregnant women were more hypnotizable than others. Of his 28 published cases, he obtained good results in 70 per cent (19 cases), ten cases had a complete analgesia, five experienced pain with the expulsion of the head, and four had their pains diminished. The eight failures were hysterical or psychopathic women, who, contrary to the usual opinion, were less hypnotizable than normal women. The criteria for assessing pain diminution were based on the opinions of the woman herself and of the midwife and doctor.

KIRSTEIN [267] of Marburg followed the Heidelberg group. He considered that at least four preparatory sessions for hypnosis were necessary. No more than three treatments a week should be given; daily treatments diminished, rather than enhanced suggestibility. His results were poorer than those of the Heidelberg group. Even in the better cases (ten) the patients groaned slightly. Amongst the remainder (eight) some cried out during the contractions, remaining calm between; the others, whom he classed as failures, woke up. He does not mention, however, how they behaved. Kirstein explained his comparatively poor results as a failure of technique—he was not present between the time when the patient was put to sleep and the delivery. During this period, the suggestions were repeated by the midwife. This was criticized by Schultze-Rhonhof who considered that the practice of the suggestive technique should be confined to the medical profession. In those cases where hypnosis proved insufficient Kirstein, following Bonne, Guckel and Friedlander, resorted to chloroform in small doses, according to the procedure of hypnonarcosis. He also dealt with the problem of analgesia versus amnesia, which he considered unsolved.

HALLAUER [217] of Berlin is reluctant to use hypnosis in its usual form, which he considers as an untimely intervention. He described his own method of narcohypnosis, in which he began the induction of hypnosis by giving small doses of chloroform. Communication between doctor and patient continued. No previous preparation was given. FLOEL [161] of Munich, used suggestion in the waking state to enhance his authority and his good relationship with the patient. At the same time he suggested that the pain of the contractions would be diminished when they came on, and in the intervals between contractions, with one hand he felt the pulse, and rested the other on the woman's abdomen.*

After 1923 the publications became more infrequent. FRANKE [171] of Breslau wrote that analgesia and amnesia were two ways in which hypnosis acted: they could occur either separately or concurrently. Another paper appeared in 1927, by VON WOLFF [578] of Berlin. The majority of the women he had delivered under hypnosis were restless during the stage of dilatation, even opening their eyes. They often maintained that they had felt no pain. Nevertheless, on account of their postpartum amnesia he considered that they had always been hypnotized. Hypnosis, according to von Wolff did not abolish vegetative pain, but its cortical perception. Restless behaviour did not indicate pain and suffering. He compared the cries of women in childbirth to those of sleepers, or of persons under drug narcosis.

A good deal later, in 1950, TRUMMLER [540] of Leipzig, took up again the work on hypnosis in obstetrical analgesia, and presented a study of 21 women. Out of these, 14 were success-

---

*JOIRE [253], of Lille, used a similar technique.

ful and six failures, with one doubtful case. Four of the failures were due to faulty techniques. The women were delivered in a hypnotic state, which, according to the author, was not equivalent to unconsciousness. At the moment of birth they were made to open their eyes and at the same time their attention was focused on the first cry of the child.

CHAPTER 6

HYPNOSUGGESTIVE METHODS IN RUSSIA AFTER 1923

ANIMAL hypnosis had been studied in Russia about 1880 by DANILEVSKI [110]—in man the first work was that of TOKARSKI [538] and BECHTEREW [35], the latter a pupil of Charcot and of Bernheim. In the foreword to the French translation of his book *Suggestion and its Role in Social Life*, Bechterew described how his researches had been inspired by the French masters, in particular by Charcot and Bernheim. 'In presenting his work to the attention of French scientists, the author would consider himself happy if it could be of use in the country which first attempted to uncover the mysteries of hypnosis and suggestion.' Hypnosis was used in obstetrics on several occasions at the beginning of the twentieth century, following the French work. (BOTKINE [55], MATVEEV [351], WIAZEMSKY [576, 577], DOBROVOLSKY [129], SEMIANNIKOV [504].)

PLATONOV, a pupil of Bechterew, began his work after the First World War. He created the Kharkov School of Psychotherapy, which laid the first foundations of the practical application of hypnosis in obstetrics. Platonov and his followers were inspired by studies already published at the end of the nineteenth century, especially by French doctors,* and more recently by the German work between 1920–1923. However, the investigations carried out in France and Germany had been given up fairly early. The Russian workers have shown a greater persistence and an enthusiasm which even led them to believe in the possibility of a mass application of hypnosuggestive methods in obstetrical analgesia. Their outlook did not prove feasible, but in any case, they showed that hypnosis was a valuable research tool in the field of psychological analgesia. It will be seen later that their experiments paved

---

*As is shown in their studies by numerous and detailed quotations from French authors who have been almost completely forgotten in France.

the way for the elaboration of the psychoprophylactic method. They cast light on its various stages as well as on those of all the other psychosomatic methods, and give their views on the many points still under discussion relating both to the theory and practice of these methods. The most instructive data will therefore be reported here.

Three periods can be distinguished in the history of hypnosuggestive methods in the USSR since 1923. The first, from 1923 to 1930, directly follows the German studies. The second, from 1936 to 1941, corresponds to a wave of interest throughout the country, in the general problem of obstetrical analgesia; and, lastly, after World War II, the hypnosuggestive method continues to be studied at various institutions.

As early as 1923, PLATONOV [426] considered that hypnosuggestive analgesia brought advantages both to the mother and to the child: decreased pains, the suppression of useless exertions for the mother and of the noxious effects of toxic substances on the child. The Kharkov psychiatrist had to fight against the disbelief and opposition of medical circles and of public opinion, and therefore carried out his first experiments on the women doctors and medical students around him. He dedicated himself to his investigations as though these were an apostolate in which he associated the women who had helped him. Of them he said 'they started their medical career gloriously. For the patient's sake, primarily, and for the triumph of scientific truth, as a vanguard they entered a field where the atmosphere was loaded with doubt, distrust and irony. . .'.

In addition to his own thanks he expressed to these same women the gratefulness of those who, delivered by this new method, 'fulfil a normal and magnificent act with a quiet smile on their lips rather than with tears in their eyes, writhing and sobbing in useless pain'.

The first woman prepared by PLATONOV was delivered by CHESTOPAL on 1 November 1923. Childbirth took place in the waking state. Analgesia was induced by post-hypnotic suggestion and the perineum was sutured without any drug anaesthesia. PLATONOV and CHESTOPAL both attended the childbirth. The parturient woman, a primiparous thirty-two year old medical student, gave a detailed account of preparation and delivery. Her self-observation* is an interesting document illuminating a living experience of hypnotic analgesia. In January 1924 the Second Congress of Russian Neuro-psychiatrists in Leningrad, PLATONOV and his pupil, VELVOVSKI, were the first to present a communication on hypnosuggestive analgesia in surgery, gynaecology, obstetrics and stomatology (three obstetrical cases) [428].

In 1925, PLATONOV and CHESTOPAL together published a booklet in which Platonov presented a tentative theoretical explanation of hypnosis based on the theories of Pavlov. The childbirth and the self-observation of the student previously mentioned were reported in the same booklet [429].

In 1927 PLATONOV described, in a communication delivered at the Gynaecological Section of the Kharkov Scientific Association, how he had 94 deliveries carried out with the hypnosuggestive method. He stressed the importance of psychotherapy in gynaecology and obstetrics, and maintained that every obstetrician should be familiar with psychotherapy, thus enabling him to free women of the fear of childbirth and of pain which have 'falsely been called physiological' [421].

About 1923, a Kiev obstetrician, NICOLAIEV, also began to investigate the use of hypnosis in gynaecology and obstetrics. NICOLAIEV mentioned the successful use of hypnosis for postoperative sedation, intractable vomiting and functional gynaecological disorders. He obtained excellent results in the cure of vaginismus; under the influence of treatment 'the woman's psyche was transformed and she often came back to life when she had been on the verge of suicide' [383].

Referring to analgesia, NICOLAIEV declared that he could remove the adenoids of a thirteen-year-old boy under hypnosis. As to obstetrical analgesia, he treated his first case in March 1923. The second stage of delivery took place under hypnosis. Aware of the shortcomings of this technique he began to use analgesia through

*The self-observations of a subject are important means of studying the experience, as it is lived through, of the hypnotic state. We are familiar with the interesting self-observations of the famous psychiatrist Eugen Bleuler, reproduced by Forel under the title *The Hypnotized Hypnotizer*.

More recently, the American psychoanalysts, BRENMAN, GILL and KNIGHT [61] using the analytical hypothesis of the ego with regard to hypnosis noted the importance of the subject's self-estimation for the study of the depth of the trance.

post-hypnotic suggestion, delivery taking place in the waking state. He reported six cases, including two failures, that he attributed to the absence of preparation. All these cases concerned women doctors or medical students. In a later study, published in 1926, NICOLAIEV declared himself in favour of the procedure of post-hypnotic suggestion. He considered that Kogerer's technique was excellent (he himself had employed it without being aware of the studies of the Viennese psychiatrist)* because, except for pain, the woman retains all subjective sensations related to childbirth. According to him, it was 'the most rational, ethical and inoffensive method' [384].

In 1927 NICOLAIEV [385] published an important paper on the 'Theory and practice of hypnosis from the physiological point of view'. This publication is interesting because it reflects the ideas current at that time, following the school of reflexology, on the theory and practice of hypnosis. Several especially significant facts may be picked out: with regard to technique, we note a certain reappraisal of mesmeric passes, with a physiological explanation for them: hypnosis, based on cortical inhibition, is obtained by stimulation. The author stresses the hierarchy of stimuli: the most effective are thermal skin stimuli, then tactile

---

*DONIGUEVITCH [132] questions the priority of the use of post-hypnotic analgesia by Kogerer. 'In fact', he said, 'as early as 1923, independently from Kogerer, this method was successfully used by Platonov, in Kharkov and by Nicolaiev in Kiev'. Incidentally, we should remember that, Kogerer's studies began in 1922, and that even if Nicolaiev claims that his own investigations are original, he does not give them any priority over those of the Viennese psychiatrist. The same applies to Platonov. The latter declared that he had practised hypnosuggestive analgesia independently of the German studies. When he became aware of the latter (which he quoted in his communication of January 1924), he felt strengthened in his decision to investigate more searchingly the medical applications of hypnosis. As has been seen, LIÉBAULT of Nancy had already raised the problem of analgesia through post-hypnotic suggestion at the end of the last century. Doniguevitch also claims for his country priority, not only for a psychotherapeutic technique in obstetrics, but for psychotherapy in general. 'In comparing the importance of Pavlov's work with that of psychotherapy abroad, we must recognize that our country is the home of a truly scientific psychotherapy. The history of psychotherapy did not begin with Mesmer, Charcot or Bernheim, but with the great Pavlov'.

stimuli, and finally auditory stimuli. The passes are regarded as thermal stimuli when applied at a certain distance from the skin, and as tactile stimuli when there is a contact. NICOLAIEV introduced 'luminous' passes, produced by a blue lamp, and which he regarded as thermal stimuli, light also favouring inhibition.*

Whatever the importance granted to mechanical stimulation, nonetheless it must be admitted that he uses verbal suggestion in explaining to the subject the sensations that will be produced by the stimuli. (Explanation given prior to hypnotization and between the passes.)

In addition, Nicolaiev warns against too many sessions. As Pavlov showed, when conditioned stimuli are too frequently repeated, they lose their efficiency more rapidly than when reproduced at longer intervals.

In the chapter called 'Hypnosis and Psychoanalysis' Nicolaiev attempts to make a synthesis between psychoanalysis and reflexology in the form of hypno-analysis. The pathogenic 'strangulated affect' is a pathologic conditioned reflex which could not be expressed, and which leaves 'associative links' in the cortex. Hypnosis is beneficial for the abreaction of the affect, because an inhibited cortex is more open and hypermnesic. If the affect is not abreacted in the cortex, it goes into unconsciousness, i.e. it does not completely disappear, but maintains certain associative links, which disturb normal cortical activity. Nicolaiev thought that it was useless for the efficacy of psychotherapy to resort to subjectivism, inevitably linked to psychoanalytic 'divination', and to use the 'nebulous' words of repression and unconsciousness. He quoted Lifchitz, according to whom six months to two years are required to discover with psychoanalysis an infantile trauma dating back to the second year of life, whereas only two to forty sessions of hypnoanalysis are necessary.†

*Luminous passes are considered by Ivanov-Smolenski as visual stimuli (quoted by ZDRAVOMYSLOV) [582]. We must note that some American workers are again using mesmeric passes by interpreting their value in a psycho-dynamic approach. KLEMPERER, for instance, considers that a light stroke on the head favours sleep because it produces memories of childhood [270].

†In the United States during the last few years authors with a psychoanalytical background have also tried to shorten therapy, by using hypnosis with psychodynamic concepts.

NICOLAIEV also considers that the indications for hypnosis were more numerous than those for psychoanalysis. He advises the teaching of hypnology in the medical schools along with physiology, neuro-psychiatry and other subjects, and regrets the limitations imposed at that time (1927) on the use of hypnosis by the Ministry of Health. It was allowed only in State-controlled therapeutic institutions and investigation centres. Its use in private clinics was submitted to special authorization: the doctor practising hypnosis had to be trained in neuro-psychiatry for at least five years. A third person had to attend the hypnotic session. Thus, NICOLAIEV said, most practitioners were deprived of a useful therapeutic tool. The author had used hypnosis in obstetrical analgesia in twenty cases: even when analgesia was not complete, the woman was quiet, disciplined and freed from fear, an undoubted advantage.

In Leningrad, the obstetrician GUERENSTEIN, a pupil of Skrobanski, was influenced by psychoanalysis and interested in psychotherapy, the use of which he propagated in obstetrics and gynaecology. In his first paper published in 1924 [209], he used psychotherapy in the treatment of gynaecological disorders, which as shown by 'the works of Bleuler, Freud and his followers' are 'in direct relation to the activity of genitality'.

As regards analgesia he reported numerous cases of curettage and a podalic version followed by removal of the foetus was carried out under hypnotic anaesthesia. A colporraphy and a total hysterectomy were also performed under a similar anaesthesia. Drug narcosis had been absolutely contraindicated in these two patients. Moreover, a Caesarian section was carried out before any sign that labour had begun, in a patient with mitral disease [209].

In a second publication (1925) GUERENSTEIN [210] studied the problem of the treatment of intractable vomiting of pregnancy and of vaginismus by psychotherapy. Whilst taking into account the somatic component of vomiting he drew attention to the psychological factors, using psychoanalytic concepts. He referred to Freud, for whom 'every hysterical symptom has its meaning'. If the patient was afraid or rejected her pregnancy, vomiting could appear as a defensive reflex 'in the shape of an unconscious reaction to the unwished-for pregnancy'. He treated the vomiting by direct suggestion under hypnosis, or by psychotherapy in the waking state in order to get insight. He described several cases where bringing back to consciousness the link between the traumatic situation and the symptom had led to the resolution of the latter.

KALACHNIK, an assistant at the Psychiatric clinic of Odessa, began to practise obstetrical hypnosis in 1925, and published in 1927 [260]. He refers to the work of the Heidelberg School and to that of Professor Platonov, who adapted the German techniques. Hypnotic suggestion was used either alone, or in combination with a narcotic (hypnonarcosis [cf. p. 24] or narcohypnosis [cf. p. 28]). The parturient woman was kept in a hypnotic state during the course of her labour, or was hypnotized toward the end of labour. This technique was somewhat inconvenient psychologically because of the amnesia for the actual birth, and because of the enormous time demands made on the doctor. Kalachnik carried out hypnosis during the preparatory sessions, the delivery taking place in the waking state.

He published nine cases all with good results, always better with primiparae than with multiparae. Among his pregnant women, some were anxious, and complained of insomnia or pains in the back. All these symptoms disappeared during the period of preparation. The women wrote down their impressions. All were delivered in a waking state. One woman alone described a state of somnolence, without loss of contact with her surroundings, following on the suggestion of analgesia made by her attending doctor.

PYRSKII [442] used psychotherapy of all types in obstetrics and gynaecology—rational psychotherapy (DUBOIS [136]), suggestion in a waking state* and under hypnosis, and psychoanalytically oriented therapy.

He praised hypnosis particularly, for by its use he obtained either a total or a partial analgesia, whilst the patient remained calm and tranquil. Delivery took place under hypnosis or in a waking state. POSTOLNIK [433], of Kiev, had since 1928 developed an extempore technique of analgesia produced by post hypnotic suggestion, the woman being delivered in a waking state. No

*Pyrskii considered that suggestion in a waking state was very close to the method used by Dubois. The latter had the opposite view [136].

preliminary preparation was given. Hypnosis was given in a general labour ward, often even amidst disturbed women in childbirth. It was administered at the request of the woman when the pains became very strong.* Visual fixation and verbal suggestion were used; three sessions were given during childbirth, in the first, calmness was suggested, in the others analgesia. He obtained good results, although his experience was limited. He himself carried out the deliveries.

In 1930, S. CHLIFER, a pupil of Platonov published her dissertation on the verbal analgesia of childbirth [92]. For her, this kind of analgesia is 'a question of neuropsychological prophylaxis and of hygiene for the mother and the foetus'. Verbal action is of capital importance. She quoted the German author Siegel, who even when he performs analgesia under the form of Dämmerschlaf, enhances the action of drugs by suggestion. The psycho-genetic factor in the pain of delivery is very important. Chlifer agrees with Lipmann's opinion that women have a special biological and psychological constitution characterized by an emotional concentration on the genitality, and a feeling of inferiority.†

This emotional concentration may in certain cases, exaggerate the pain of childbirth and, in others, suppress it. The existence of naturally painless delivery is well known.

Another proof of the importance of the psychological factor is shown in the influence of environment on the 'neuro-psychic'

*This is an important point, because the women believed in the analgesic efficacy of the procedure.

†These two ideas on the female constitution are the result of two trends of thought at that time. On the one hand, there is a remnant of the ancient conception of hysteria, a woman's disease 'par excellence'. This conception was strongly disputed by Charcot and Freud. On the other hand, there is an echo of Freud's 'androcentric' ideas he had stressed the 'claim for masculinity' as a factor of neurosis in women. It is interesting to note that, on the contrary, several authors have emphasized man's concentration on the uro-genital sphere. For instance, Jules Janet (1890) a famous urologist of that time and brother of Pierre Janet, wrote that only men are affected with 'urinary hypochondria', because women perfectly understand the possibility of coitus, despite lesions of the bladder and urethra.

With Aboulker and Muriel Cahen we have investigated psychosomatic uro-genital pain, and seen, as was expected, that both sexes were affected.

constitution: peasant women and primitive women have an easier delivery than others.

The author quoted BOUKOMSKI who reported the painless childbirth of a drunken woman. She herself relates the case of a twenty-nine-year-old student with a contracted pelvis who, being in prison, had a painless childbirth after being told that she was threatened with a death sentence. CHLIFER experimented with the various kinds of hypnosuggestive method. She came out in favour of analgesia by post-hypnotic suggestion, so that an act as important in a woman's life as childbirth should not take place outside the realm of consciousness.

The analgesia is not proportional to the depth of hypnosis obtained during the preparation, and good results can be obtained even by suggestion in the waking state. Extemporary preparation is also possible. The author was led to an interesting observation, stressing the importance of inter-personal relationship in hypnosuggestive analgesia: her mere presence with the women she had prepared had an analgesiant effect. 'My personal experience enables me to say,' she wrote, 'that the success of verbally induced analgesia is closely related to the personality of the subject and the relationship established between the doctor and the parturient woman'. CHLIFER gave a tentative reflexological explanation of this relationship. The hypnotizer must be considered as a 'combined conditional stimulus' which corresponds to a strictly differentiated reaction in the subject's cortex. She gave, as evidence, the experiment of PLATONOV who managed to condition a subject so that he failed to feel an electric current in the presence of a given person. Finally the importance of the doctor–patient relationship is further demonstrated by the special attention given by the author to the initial interview during which the relationship is established. She quoted DÉJERINE who considers that the success of psychotherapy for psychoneurosis depended on the initial interview.*

BOJOVSKI and TOUREVSKI of Tumen [51], while 'thinking that pain binds the mother to the child somatically and psychologically and arouses her maternal instinct' considered that it, in many

---

*The problem of the 'initial interview' is being investigated at present in the U.S.A. with a psychoanalytic approach. A book on this subject has been published by a research group at Yale University.

cases, was useless. They advised an individual approach and declared themselves in favour of the hypnosuggestive method, which they used in thirty-three cases. GUEORGUIEVSKI of Nijni-Novgorod [208] also practised the method and thought that, at that time, it was used by some thirty practitioners in the USSR. As early as 1912 he used hypnosis in obstetrics and could regulate the rhythm of uterine contractions by suggestions. In 1925, another Moscow obstetrician, ZDRAVOMYSLOV, began his work in this field. He published his first paper in 1930 [582]; it will be discussed in detail later. During that period, IOFFE in Dniepropetrovsk, KOUDACHEV in Kazan, ISTOMINE, KISLOV, MOTSAK and MILOSLAVSKI in Kharkov and GOURSTEIN in Oufa, should also be mentioned.

For several years, the number of investigations into the hypnosuggestive method was reduced, but since 1936 there has again been a renewed interest in its favour. In 1936 PLATONOV analysed the results of 588 cases treated by him and his associates, most women being delivered in the waking state. In 60 per cent of these cases a good result was obtained. He drew attention to the importance of the doctor–patient relationship, the rate of complete success being higher when the operator was present at childbirth. Platonov stressed that even in pregnant women who had no analgesia, the preparation produced a general strengthening effect and the disappearance of pathological somatic and psychologic reactions such as dyspepsia, nausea, vomiting, signs of toxaemia...

These beneficial effects were seen in 95 per cent of the pregnant women. In addition, the preparation permitted the discovery of neurotic symptoms, and psychotherapy could be applied. Platonov's pupils also experimented with extemporary preparation. Its efficacy was linked to the presence of the operator during delivery. Platonov also emphasized the fact that psychotherapy must accompany drug-induced analgesia itself. Lastly he advised a thorough psychotherapeutic education for the nursing and medical staff, with lectures and interviews about 'special psychoprophylaxis'. All obstetricians certainly do not have this psychotherapeutic understanding, and Platonov declared 'It is essential that the negative and ironic attitude at present shown by obstetricians toward the psychotherapeutic method, as we have observed it do during the present study, should disappear'.

In 1940, PLATONOV studied the problem of indirect suggestion and suggestion linked to the administration of drugs. He reported the investigations of his collaborators Tsvetkov and Proniavieva who obtained nearly the same analgesic effects with placebos as with drugs (veronal, chloral, magnesium sulphate). Analgesia induced by cupping on Head's areas was attributed by Platonov to a purely suggestive influence. He also considered that the psychologic effect may give a therapeutic value to an indifferent product, or increase the effect of a worth-while drug. In addition, the same product will display different effects according to the therapists using them, because 'there is a dynamic relationship between the types of higher nervous activities of two people, the doctor and his patient'.

The obstetrician TSVETKOV [542] used direct suggestion without preparation, referring to the studies of Le Menant de Chesnais who, according to him, was the first to use this technique. He fought against the erroneous belief that suggestion would be ineffective on women not prepared over a long period, and successfully prepared, extemporaneously, 68 women. Suggestion was made in the waking state in 54 cases and in a somnolent state in 14. Here are the main points of his technique: a good relationship is established with the parturient woman when she is admitted to the maternity hospital. She becomes acquainted, as much as possible, with women delivered without pain by the hypnosuggestive method or drug-induced analgesia. Later, she is given suggestion between contractions, either by the Bernheim–Bechterew procedure (awake, and her eyes closed, she is given direct suggestions of analgesia) or by the Loewenfeld–Bechterew procedure (identical with the former, but the woman is in a state of somnolence). For this technique, the continuous presence of the doctor during childbirth is mandatory. He carries out 'invigorating' interviews with the parturient woman between contractions.

Another collaborator of Platonov, KOPIL-LEVINA, a psychiatrist, in 1940 published the results of a five-year investigation [278]. She seeks to simplify the hypnosuggestive method, to render it practicable for obstetricians, who ought, however, to familiarize themselves with psychotherapy. The simplest type is direct suggestion, including short statements, imperative orders, and affirmations, without any active participation or critical attitude on the part of the subject. Another form of elementary suggestion is indirect suggestion, consisting in the administration of indifferent products claimed to be analgesic. KOPIL-LEVINA does not want to restrict herself to this elementary suggestion, and she introduces more elaborate forms of psychotherapy, the 'motivated' suggestion and 'rational' psychotherapy of Dubois, of Berne. In 'motivated' suggestion, the subject has a passive attitude but the doctor adds to suggestion elements of education, persuasion and reassurance. After inquiring into the psychological history of the subject, she gives explanations to reassure her as to the cause of her worries and anxieties.

Dubois' 'rational' psychotherapy represents, for Kopil-Levina, the most elaborate form of psychotherapy. It includes all elements mentioned above, stress being laid on the need for the doctor to convince the patient that her fears are not justified; in addition the patient must adopt an active attitude during the 'analytical' interview with the doctor as well as in her fight against her difficulties. Kopil-Levina considers that the Coué method may sometimes be useful as an auxiliary.

Psychotherapy will be carried out in the waking state during the interviews; sometimes the Bernheim–Bechterew method will be used for direct and 'motivated' suggestion. These two forms of suggestion may also be used in a state of slight hypnosis (Lowenfeld–Bechterew procedure). In addition, suggested sleep will be resorted to in sessions of 'hypnosis-rest' to obtain the beneficial effect of the hypnotic state itself. The author recommends that detailed information on the course of childbirth, its physiological nature, on the suppression of fear, and of negative emotions be given during the interviews. Letters from mothers delivered by the method may be read, or the subjects may even be put in touch with them. Kopil-Levina emphasizes the qualities the doctor must show: benevolence, firmness, assurance, faith in the method, spirit of initiative etc. . . . The success of the method will also depend on the relationship of sympathy and trust established between the doctor and the parturient woman.

In 1936 NICOLAIEV spoke at the Second Congress of Obstetricians and Gynaecologists of the Donetz area. He stated that the first stage of delivery is the most painful, because the woman is passive, whereas she is active in the second stage. No analgesic drug seemed satisfactory to him, and he deplored the lack of objective criteria for assessing the degree of analgesia. In his opinion, the hypno-suggestive method had the disadvantages of requiring a long preparation, and a favourable atmosphere, which is not always easy to find. He had given up the method temporarily since 1926 [386]. In 1936 NICOLAIEV also published a more important study, in which he re-examined the suggestive method of obstetrical analgesia. 'This method', he wrote, 'should be generally applied, and be amongst the first group of analgesic methods, because it gives the best results, has the greatest physiological action, does not introduce any biologically active chemical into the body, and is not dangerous for the mother and the child' [387]. He stressed the major role of the thalamus in the production of pain, 'the pain of childbirth being essentially a protopathic, thalamic pain'. Nicolaiev also laid emphasis on direct and indirect suggestion, the atmosphere of the maternity hospital being an important factor in indirect suggestion. He modified his technique of hypnotization, concentrating on the visual stimulation of the subject. This was on the basis of a theory in vogue at that time according to which fatigue of the ocular muscles, after transmission to the diencephalic nuclei, would act on the contiguous sleep centre. Nicolaiev also stressed the advantages of analgesia by means of post-hypnotic suggestion, because, thanks to this technique, 'the woman takes an active part in childbirth'. He considered preparation to be very important, and questioned the efficacy of extemporary intervention.

The most important work of the period was that of KATCHAN and BELOZERSKI [262] on the 'Method of selection for obstetrical analgesia by hypnosuggestion'. It covers 501 cases including 369 primiparae and 132 multiparae. This long study, the essential points of which are given here, was originally designed to solve the problem of the selection of pregnant women in relation to the method and its variants. The following controversial questions were dealt with: analgesic efficacy; the relationship between analgesia and amnesia; the most favourable time to begin the preparation; the number of sessions; the depth of trance; the influence of the method on the mother and the child; the results other than analgesia; and the possibility of delivery in the waking state.

The authors selected women according to the following criteria: suggestibility and hypnotizability: ability to carry out post-hypnotic suggestions; the state of health of the pregnant woman with special reference to the nervous system; presence or absence of fear related to childbirth; sensibility to pain; period of pregnancy or delivery at which preparation was started.

Hypnotizability was assessed according to the three usual stages: the first corresponding to slight hypnosis, the hypnotized subject being able to resist suggestions and to open the eyes; the second corresponding to deeper sleep, with spontaneous and suggested catalepsy and analgesia; the third corresponding to deep hypnosis, and the possible production of hallucinations and partial amnesia. Suggestibility could be good, fair, weak or very weak, according to Birman's test or to Astakhov's test.*

Seven variants of the method were chosen by the authors:

1. Individual preparation, with analgesia induced by post-hypnotic suggestion;
2. Collective preparation with analgesia induced by post-hypnotic suggestion;
3. Use of hypnosis during delivery, without preparation;
4. Individual preparation and childbirth under hypnosis (1 and 3);
5. Collective preparation and delivery under hypnosis (2 and 3);
6. Hypno-narcosis;
7. Narco-hypnosis.

On the basis of their criteria of hypnotizability and suggestibility, the authors distinguished five groups of women:

I. Good suggestibility and third stage of hypnosis;

II. Good suggestibility and second stage at the first session; third stage obtained before the third session;

III. Less good suggestibility and second stage at the fourth session;

IV. Weak suggestibility and second stage of hypnosis;

---

*In Birman's test the subject closes his eyes, his forehead is gently touched with a reflex hammer, and he is told that he cannot open his eyes. In Astakhov's test, the same suggestion is made, but pressure is exerted on the eyeballs (cf. p. 137).

V. Poor suggestibility and first stage of hypnosis with no increase during the course of preparation.

The best results were obtained in the following order: method 5, 2, 1, 4 and 3. In group I, all methods good; in group II, a long preparation is necessary; in groups III and IV, a collective preparation is required and delivery should be performed under hypnosis; in group V, no satisfactory results are achieved by hypnosis.

Table of Results

Methods	Total No. of cases	No.	%	No.	%	No.	%	No.	%	Positive Results No.	%
1	63	37	59	15	24	1	2	10	15	52	83
2	51	25	49	22	43	—	—	4	8	47	92
3	59	30	51	17	29	3	5	9	15	47	80
4	16	11	69	2	12	—	—	3	9	13	81
5	16	9	56	6	38	—	—	1	6	15	94
6	215	15	7	93	43	47	22	60	28	108	50
7	81	19	23	37	46	9	11	16	20	56	69
	501	56	29	192	38	60	12	103	21	338	67

Table of Prognosis

Groups	Agreement No.	%	Disagreement Sup. Results		Inf. Results.	
I	7	35	6	30	7	35
II	7	35	12	60	1	5
III	3	15	15	75	2	10
IV	4	20	14	70	2	10
V	5	25	14	70	1	5
	26	26	61	61	13	13

The first method is indicated for groups I and II, the second for groups I, II and III; the third for groups I and II; the fourth for groups III and IV; the fifth for groups IV and, partially V; the sixth and seventh for group V. The results were as above (see Table). Complete analgesia was obtained in 29 per cent of the cases; partial analgesia in 38 per cent. Doubtful results were seen in 12 per cent and failure in 21 per cent.

For the whole group of women, positive results were obtained in 67 per cent (or 65 per cent in primiparae, and 73 per cent in multiparae). Katchan and Belozersky explained that their results were inferior to those of other authors and, especially, of the Heidelberg School (90-100 per cent) due to the fact that the latter authors had included in their statistics only parturient women treated with methods 4 and 5. The results obtained by Katchan and Belozerski with these methods were also positive in 90-100 per cent of the cases.

A prognosis of the results was made according to the group in which they were classified, presence or absence of fear, sensitivity to pain and peculiarities of pregnancy. The results were assessed on the basis of the observations of the house doctor and of the Chief of the Unit, completed by an interrogation of the mother lasting one hour, several days and several months after childbirth. Prognosis was made on groups of twenty women (see Table).

On the whole, prognosis and results were in agreement in 26 per cent of the cases, prognosis was inferior to results in 61 per cent and superior in 13 per cent.

In conclusion, the authors considered that a careful selection of the pregnant women for this or that method conditions the quality of the results; the latter will also depend on the depth of the trance obtained in the sessions of preparation, and on good suggestibility. The deeper the trance obtained, the better the suggestibility, the more limited the number of sessions required, and the later the starting time of preparation.

If hypnosis needs to be used extempore, it is best that hypnotization take place during advanced dilatation. Analgesia or hypnotic hypoanalgesia may occur spontaneously or be the result of a suggestion acting during or following hypnosis; collective preparation increases hypnotizability and suggestibility. The efficacy of the hypnosuggestive method decreases with age, protracted delivery, exaggerated sensitivity to pain, fear related to childbirth, duration of the interval between the last sitting and delivery, unfavourable conditions of childbirth (agitation, cries of neighbours etc. . .). Amnesia does not always follow a good analgesic result.

The use of hypno-suggestive methods entails no danger for the mother and the child. Besides its analgesic effect, the hypnosuggestive method may result in the disappearance of the fear of childbirth, and may sometimes invigorate the pregnant woman. In some cases, the uterine activity can be controlled by suggestion.

After World War II, new investigations were carried out on the hypnosuggestive method. VIGDOROVITCH of Leningrad, whose studies date back to 1935, was mainly preoccupied with the mass application of the method; for this purpose, he created a 'hypnotarium', where he prepared pregnant women for their labours, which took place in different maternity clinics in the city [563]. His experience covered several thousands of cases. He prepared women collectively, grouping five, eight, 15 and even 70 of them. He conditioned women to fall asleep at the sound of a bell.

Vigdorovitch was a convinced partisan of the hypnosuggestive method, which he preferred to drug analgesia. As well as its analgesic effects, he ascribed to the method a decrease in puerperal complications and a beneficial action on lactation. Results depend much on the atmosphere of the maternity hospital and the attitude of the staff. He favoured an early rupture of the membranes, which improved the analgesic results and accelerated childbirth. SYRKINE [517] also 'prepared' 600 women in a hypnotarium in Kiev. KOGANOV has used hypnosis for obstetrical analgesia since 1935 at the Medical Institute at Kharkov, in the Clinic of Professor Chmoundak. In 1951 he published [274] a technique of extempore preparation using suggestion, either under hypnosis or in the waking state. The preparation began when the women arrived at the clinic, and delivery took place either in a hypnotic sleep or awake. Koganov conditioned the woman in such a way that the uterine contractions became the signal for the beginning of the hypnotic state. 'At the approach of a contraction, it was suggested to the woman that she closed her eyes, took a deep breath and went to sleep. Awakening took place after the finish of the contraction. . . . The wish to remain free from pain allowed a rapid establishment of a temporary link between the contractions and sleep.' Koganov writes of his experiences in 1300 cases, but only gives the results of 460.

Kogan, of Tashkent, also used suggestion to obtain obstetrical analgesia.

The most important work on these hypnosuggestive methods has been recently published by ZDRAVOMYSLOV in his book [585] entitled *Obstetrical Analgesia Produced by Suggestion*. It appeared after the official adoption of the Psychoprophylactic Method. The author considers that 'as well as analgesia produced by the Psychopropylactic Method or by pharmacological means, there are also other psychotherapeutic (suggestive) methods. The suggestive method is not opposed to the Psychoprophylactic Method, which at the present stage is the chief 'method.' This latter, 'thanks to the east and generality of application (it can even be practised by the midwife in the maternity unit of a collective farm) allows for the easing, to various degrees, of the pain of childbirth in millions of women. But its efficacy is much inferior to that of the hypnosuggestive methods.' Zdravomyslov also writes 'psychoprophylaxis of childbirth in certain cases is alone not sufficient, and therapy becomes necessary'. At that point, hypnosuggestive methods are brought into use. These methods have been used in cases where 'for one reason or another the labour was expected to be extremely painful'. In this group are women suffering from toxaemia,* serious organic disease, contracted pelvis, elderly primiparae, or those having previously experienced a very painful or pathological labour. Since 1935 he has studied 1000 cases, 700 with, and 300 without previous preparation. Of the 700, half consisted of difficult cases in whom a therapeutic approach was necessary.

Zdravomyslov added a theoretical modification to the ideas of Velvovski on reflex-conditioned pain.† He considers that there are two components to the pain: (1) 'Real pain', (the material substrate

*Women suffering from toxaemia do not necessarily suffer from a more painful labour than others.
†Cf. Chapter 9.

of pain, according to Nicolaiev) linked with the first signalling system; (2) 'Suggested pain', linked with the second signalling system (language).

He prefers the expression 'suggested pain' to that of reflex-conditioned pain, used at the Leningrad Congress in 1951. He admits that there is a reflex-conditioned pain amongst multiparae who have had a previously painful labour. But 'a conditioned reflex, in the strict sense of the word, cannot be produced in the cortices of women who have never been in labour. In these women it is possible to speak of a conditioned reflex produced by the culturally linked conviction of the inevitability of the pains of childbirth; one can conceive of an elaboration, by way of the second signalling system, of a temporary link, which may also be more permanent, between the words childbirth and pain'. According to Zdravomyslov, verbal suggestion can abolish the two types of pain.

Preparation, either individual or group (three to 20 persons) was used, and the sessions varied between one and 16 in number. Various methods were used:

(1) Preparatory hypnosuggestion. Delivery under either light or deep hypnosis, or in a waking state; the therapist was present throughout or at intervals, or even absent.

(2) Hypnosuggestion without preparation, otherwise similar to (1).

(3) Suggestion alone without previous preparation.

(4) Indirect suggestion. The efficacy of this, otherwise termed 'suggestion through activity', has been confirmed by Nicolaiev, Platonov and others. Indirect suggestion in the shape of 'pain reducing procedures' was of great importance in the development of the psychoprophylactic methods.*

The patients are also given instruction into physiological mechanisms; during the preparatory period he does not only make suggestions directly relating to the pain, but also uses

---

*Zdravomyslov recommends the giving of verbal suggestion together with placebos in different forms—such as powders, drugs, injections and other substances (Kiparski chalks, etc.), recommended by PLOTITCHER [430] on the psychoprophylactic method. It is said by the latter that a cortical activation is produced by these means.

educative and psychotherapeutic measures. When the woman is under hypnosis he reassures her, speaks of physiological mechanisms, and of her behaviour during childbirth (in order to strengthen the teaching carried out in a waking state). Of primary importance is the attitude of doctor and nurse toward the hypnosuggestive method. The prestige and authority of the doctor ought to be as great as is possible, and should be upheld by the whole group dealing with the patient. The relationship between doctor and patient should be based, from the beginning, on confidence and understanding. It is important that the doctor should be present at all phases during the labour, and the results are in direct relation to this. Thus it is more rational for the obstetrician to be taught the hypnosuggestive method, so that he may practise it himself. Platonov has upheld this viewpoint since 1925.

Zdravomyslov believes that it is possible to influence the contractions by means of suggestion. His investigations were carried out with the help of the 'tokodynamometer'. Whether multiparae or primiparae respond more to the method is difficult to say. As to the relationship between the depth of the trance and the degree of analgesia, he feels that the latter increases with the former. He sees no danger in hypnosis as long as it is properly carried out, and this can be learnt by most doctors. He quotes Wetterstrand, with 60,000 hypnotic treatments to his credit without complication. On his part, over the course of 35 years, Zdravomyslov has carried out 15,000 treatments. 'We have seen nothing but good results as regards the general and moral health of the patients.'

VELVOVSKI [558] summed up the position, and considered that 8000 case reports had been published over the last 25 or 30 years.

From a theoretical point of view most authors consider the hypnosuggestive method as more or less linked with Pavlovian conceptions. Some stress this relationship, others not. Opposition to the conditioned-reflex explanation also exists.

AMFITEATROV [14], for instance writes 'It is forcing the facts to postulate that one session of 10–15 minutes, made on the day before the delivery of one or other woman, was able to form and consolidate a conditioned reflex to a word.' He mentions that Pavlov's dogs would go to sleep, at a signal in the laboratory, but not outside. On this account his patients were prepared outside the labour ward.*

These theoretical divergencies do not prevent the different authorities from reaching agreement in practice. They are unanimous on the reality of 'verbal' analgesia and this conviction led Velvovski and his associates, as we shall see later, to create the psychoprophylactic method.

The period which we have described above is rich in lessons. Interest in hypnosis lasted for a longer period than it had previously in other countries, in France for instance, the cradle of hypnosis, interest hardly outlived Charcot's death, the reason being that to his pupils the psychological explanations seemed too vague and the objective physiological data insufficient.

The Russian authors who believed in the reflexological explanation of hypnosis were, on the contrary, stimulated in their investigations. Thus, they inquired into the use of hypnosis in obstetrical analgesia with the greatest enthusiasm. In this struggle to relieve the pain of childbirth, Platonov showed a missionary spirit similar to that shown later by Read in England and Lamaze in France.

The Russian authors encountered technical difficulties in the mass application of the hypnosuggestive method. From the beginning, while performing deliveries under hypnosis, they preferred deliveries in the waking state, obtaining analgesia by post-hypnotic suggestion, which allows the woman to take part actively in her own delivery and, above all, does not require the presence of the doctor. In the second period, they developed these procedures, as well as direct and indirect suggestion in the waking state.

The third period is still marked by an attempt of mass application, with the creation of 'hypnotariums' in large cities like Leningrad and Kiev. Besides elementary suggestion, purely didactic and psychotherapeutic elements were introduced into the method at these different periods.

Despite all these efforts, a mass application of the hypnosuggestive

---

*Amfiteatrov, moreover, is a believer in parapsychology. Starting from the studies of Richet, Ochorowicz and others, he claims to have obtained obstetric analgesia with mental telepathy. In 1927, NICOLAIEV [385] admitted the possibility of mental telepathy in animals. They could be induced to carry out actions under the influence of transmitted thought. Nicolaiev considered that Lazarev's theory on the transmission of thought, in the form of electromagnetic waves, was likely. The brain of the higher animals would receive these waves and act in accordance. This hypothesis seemed to him substantiated by the experiments of various authors, including Bechterew.

method failed to take place. It is likely that the resistance which hypnosis always encounters everywhere was added to the technical difficulties. In the end, the hypnosuggestive method was replaced by the Psychoprophylactic Method, but it remained as an auxiliary method, applicablee specially in difficult cases. On the other hand, the hypnosuggestive method has demonstrated the experimental value of the hypnotic relationship, a magnified form of any psychotherapeutic relationship. The methodological difficulties inherent in the study of the psychotherapeutic relationship, both qualitatively and quantitatively, are well known. Just because it is a macroscopic form of relationship, the hypnotic relationship might help reduce these difficulties. No one can question the role of hypnosis in the history of psychotherapy, from the first discoveries of Mesmer to the birth of psychoanalysis. Theoretically, problems related to the hypnosuggestive method and to the Psychoprophylactic Method are far from being solved. Their solutions will come together. But the Russian work brings a new confirmation of the importance of interpersonal relationship in obtaining analgesia. The interpersonal relationship is the keystone of all these methods. However, by using exclusively the adjacent 'verbal', the Russian authors brought a limitation to the psychotherapeutic relationship, because the intersubjective communication is not established only by speech. As psychotherapists, Platonov and his associates must have understood that a 'meeting' of two personalities occurred, and that psychotherapeutic results will depend on intra- and interpersonal relationship. Russian authors admit the importance of personality in the form of Nervous Types, the determination of which is very difficult in man. They only take into account the Nervous Type of the pregnant woman, but that of the doctor is also important.*

Pavlov's followers have begun to study hypnosis in animals, but the resemblance between animal hypnosis and human hypnosis is questioned, because of the existence of speech in man.†

But does speech, the second signalling system, cover all interpersonal emotional relations? Pavlov himself often noted that speech as a stimulus cannot be compared either qualitatively or quantitatively to any of the other physical stimuli. By reducing to 'verbal' the emotional interpersonal relations, the Russian authors were led to use somewhat elementary or even out-dated concepts. Thus, they always use Dubois's (of Berne) 'persuasive' psychotherapy, which is considered obsolete in all other countries.

*As stressed by Tsouladze and Coenca at the Symposium held in Paris on 7 April 1957 (see p. 162) [541].

†It has been pointed out that an animal cannot carry out a post-hypnotic suggestion.

In spite of these theoretical drawbacks, we do not wish to question the practical results obtained in obstetrical analgesia by the Russian doctors, since in psychotherapy in general, and particularly at this level (hypnosuggestive method) the personality of the therapist is an element of primary importance.

In conclusion, even though this period brings us very valuable data for understanding the Psychoprophylactic Method, the theoretical problems still remain to be solved.

CHAPTER 7

THE READ METHOD

1. THEORY

GRANTLY DICK READ first described his method in his book *Natural Childbirth*, published in 1933. *Revelation of Childbirth* appeared in 1942 in Great Britain, being published in the U.S.A. in 1944 under the title of *Childbirth Without Fear, the Principles and Practices of Natural Childbirth*. The French translation of *Childbirth Without Fear* entitled *L'Accouchement sans Douleur* was published in 1953. Studies of Read's method have been published by his followers HEARDMAN [221, 222], THOMS [529–537], and GOODRICH [192–194]. What are the salient features of his method?

One day some time before 1914 he was called to a delivery in Whitechapel, a poor district in the East End of London, a call which led to a 'revelation'. The birth went according to plan, except when Read tried to give the woman some chloroform to ease her pain, and she gently but firmly refused. This puzzled him, and later when the birth was over, he asked her why she would not have the chloroform. She replied 'It didn't hurt. It wasn't meant to, was it, Doctor?' So it was that following this experience Read was led to realize that 'there was no law in nature and no design that could justify the pain of childbirth'. This idea serves as a basic postulate in all his researches. He carried them out with the enthusiasm and faith only met with in pioneers who have had to fight against the forces of scepticism. His merit was to take systematic account of the emotional factor in labour, and to define his attitude in consequence of this. 'Confidence, understanding, and absence of fear are', he says, 'the essential factors in painless childbirth'. Read undoubtedly obtained practical successes; the theoretical bases of his methods are, however, very far from being certain. They rest on the triad, fear, tension, pain.

In outline, the theory of natural childbirth is as follows: 'Civilization and culture have brought influences to bear upon the minds of women, which have introduced justifiable fears and anxieties concerning labour. The more cultured the races of the earth have become, so much the more dogmatic have they been in pronouncing childbirth to be a painful and dangerous ordeal. This fear and anticipation have given rise to natural protective tensions in the body, and such tensions are not of the mind only, for the mechanism of protective action by the body includes muscular tension. Unfortunately the natural tension produced by fear influences those muscles which close the womb and prevent the child from being driven out during childbirth. Therefore, fear inhibits: that is to say, gives rise to resistance at the outlet of the womb, when in the normal state those muscles should be relaxed and free from tension. Such resistance and tension give rise to real pain, because the uterus is supplied with organs which record pain set up by excessive tension. Therefore, fear, pain and tension are the three evils which are not normal to the natural design, but which have been introduced in the course of civilization by the ignorance of those who have been concerned with attendance at childbirth. If pain, fear and tension go hand in hand, then it must be necessary to relieve tension and to overcome fear in order to eliminate pain. The implementation of my theory is demonstrated in the methods by which fear may be overcome, tension may be eliminated and replaced by physical and mental relaxation.'

'The normal and natural result of this is that there is excessive tension, and soon the simple sensations of uterine contractions—which have been misinterpreted by the thalamus as pain—have given rise to a neuromuscular condition which actually causes real pain.'

Thus Read defines the physiological mechanism of pain production through fear. He believes that the uterine contraction is normally painless, because 'there is no physiological function in the body which gives rise to pain in the normal course of health'. How has contraction become painful? 'The sensations arising from the uterus may be influenced in the most astonishing way by the mental condition of the woman concerned. . . . A woman about to start her first labour has been told to expect certain sensations; if she has been told wisely, her expectations have not necessarily been associated with pain, but rather with new sensations. The contractions of the uterus will be a new experience to her. If, however, emotional influences have definitely increased the intensity of her interpretation of these new sensations, they may quite easily be interpreted as pain. Should that be so, the thalamus, in conjunction with the cortex, immediately sets up a protective mechanism. Now, the great protective nerve mechanism of the body is the sympathetic nervous system, and when protection is called for by the thalamus, that nervous system overrides, by its powerful influences, all other nerve stimuli throughout the body. It activates the machinery for either fight or flight; it creates a state of tension throughout the individual which provides for an increase of muscular power.' Sensitivity to pain is further reinforced by conditions such as anaemia, mental fatigue, loss of self-control or by suggestion.

Thus there was, Read believed, an original fear which resulted in a false interpretation of normal uterine contractions, and made them painful. These 'false' pains reinforced the fear, thus creating a state of neuromuscular tension, which itself gives rise to 'true' pain. As a result there are two kinds of pain, one of central origin, the other of peripheral origin, but the association which Read establishes between them does not seem to have been proved neurophysiologically. What then is the genesis of the fear? Read at one moment speaks of fear, at another of unconscious fear which has become second nature; yet again of individuals who are a prey to anxiety, who in reality are not threatened by a real danger, but by the mental elaboration of certain hypotheses, which are exaggerated by the imagination. It is difficult to assign one identical cause to the many different forms of fear, and to bring them all under the same aegis. For example whilst speaking of the imagination, Read does not appear to include all the psychoaffective complexes which this word covers and which can exercise an effect on the intensity of the pain of childbirth. Read wants to see the fear only as a product of civilization, which carries with it preconceived ideas as to the pain of delivery. These ideas are to be found in the mother's talks to her daughter, her sisters' conversation, in newspapers and magazines, novels, and literature in general. They are enhanced by doctors and midwives. Finally women's ignorance with regard to the whole matter of childbirth itself adds to the fear to which they are and will be exposed.

2. PRACTICE

Three elements are essential in the practice of Read and his followers Heardman, Thoms and Goodrich.

(a) Didactic Methods

These consist of teaching the woman anatomical and physiological facts relating to the act of childbirth.

(b) Physiotherapeutic Methods

The principal method used is relaxation. The patient is taught to contract the different muscle groups in such a way as to feel the tension in them, and then to feel the 'letting go'. The authors recommend the technique of 'progressive relaxation' as described by JACOBSON [246], although Jacobson himself criticizes them for what he considers a false interpretation of his work. Relaxation is practised during the contractions from the stage of two-finger dilatation to that of complete dilatation (or intermediary stage). In this latter stage, not every woman is able to carry out relaxation. In the expulsive phase the woman ought to carry out relaxation between the contractions. For Read body relaxation must be recognized as a 'necessary phenomenon'; it ought to be accompanied by a mental indifference to the uterine contraction. Heardman speaks of two forms of relaxation: mental relaxation and physical relaxation. The first corresponds to a simple state of repose adopted in the interval between contractions in the phase of dilatation. The second is, for her, true relaxation, neuro-muscular relaxation. This physical relaxation, or conscious relaxation ought to be used carefully because, Goodrich writes, 'as paradoxical as this may seem, it can become fatiguing because it involves concentration'.* Antenatal exercises are practised 'to ensure that the change of shape necessitated by the increased size of the abdomen during the later months of pregnancy does not result in muscle weakness, bad position or lack of tone in those structures the efficiency of which is of importance in normal childbirth' (Read).

*CHOUGOM [93], in Russia, gives the same advice concerning the use of pain reducing procedures in the psychoprophylactic method. The thoeretical consequences which this implies will be discussed later (cf. p. 126).

On the other hand in *Antenatal Illustrated* (1955), READ recommends the 'demonstration and practice of correct breathing so that the mother may be in good fettle and the unborn baby well-nourished as it grows in the womb. One of the life-lines of the baby is in the mother's breathing' [464].

In the same work Read recommends four respiratory exercises: (1) Deep respiration; (2) more rapid respiration—from twenty-five to twenty-six respirations a minute. The exercise should be practised during the contractions, at the phase of advanced dilatation; this type of respiration is of much help in labour during a contraction* (3 and 4). These two exercises ought to help the woman in the expulsive period. One consists in holding the breath for as long as possible and the other in making short, panting respirations at about 35–40 per minute.

Read's followers attach equal importance to respiratory exercises, of which they describe different varieties, but give very little explanation as to the mechanism of their action. They particularly stress that the exercises ought to facilitate relaxation. At the phase of complete dilatation they use lumbar massage as an analgesic. This can be given, in certain cases, by the husband.

(c) *Psychotherapeutic Methods*

These are implicit in the first two groups of methods, both of which diminish pain by familiarizing the pregnant woman with the processes of childbirth, and by creating an atmosphere of confidence. Everything in the method is directed to the suppression of fear, and Read stresses as most essential the establishment of a good relationship between the doctor and the patient. As to suggestion itself, Read considers that it is 'the greatest and most harmless anaesthetizing agent that we have', a 'weapon' with which all obstetricians ought to be equipped. He considers that the term itself has been grossly abused—'Even today it is the ultimate explanation of the ignorant man for phenomena which he wishes to appear to understand'. 'Every good physician depends for success,' says Read, 'upon the correct diagnosis, his patient's faith and his conscious or unconscious powers of suggestion.' As to the mode of action of suggestion, which is very far from being

---

*This exercise, with its justification, seems to have been introduced over the last few years.

explained, it does not seem to be difficult for Read. The suggestion deals with the subconscious, which, 'not being subject to the trials of discretion, reason, discrimination, argument or logic, accepts blindly the statement made, and so long as interference by the conscious brain is kept out, so long the "suggestion" maintains power and action'. At the phase of advanced dilatation there clearly exists a lowering of the activity of the conscious mind. This is the propitious moment to give suggestions. Moreover Read stresses that suggestion can occupy a large part of the interpersonal relationship when he writes 'the obstetrician who scorns the use of mental reinforcement has overlooked that by his actions, thoughts and sympathies he has unwittingly applied the most powerful suggestion'. The whole atmosphere of maternity hospitals, the labour ward with its shining instruments, glass cases, and sterility also exert an unfavourable suggestive effect, which it is necessary to counteract by positive suggestions. Education, which struggles against the evils of false suggestion, that is to say the inherited prejudices of civilization, ought to be enhanced by the use of suggestion 'as a means of infiltrating the subconscious with truth'.

Having thus described the action of suggestion, Read takes up the question of hypnosis. He warns against confusing suggestion with hypnosis. It may be that basically they have something in common but 'the depth of influence is different'. This antagonism with regard to hypnosis is constantly found in Read's writings. Thus when he speaks of the beginning of his work he writes, 'I do not hesitate to record that so startling were the results of this teaching when I first employed it in the practice of natural childbirth, that I became suspicious of myself, although I was aware that no conscious effort was being made to influence the minds of my patients by suggestion or hypnotism. Consequently I consulted one of the greatest authorities upon these subjects, and asked him to examine me and my methods to see whether, by some accident, I was unwittingly employing the use of methods of which I was unconscious. I have never had any knowledge of mesmerism or hypnotism. The examination was most carefully made, and I was assured that there was no relation whatever between the application of relaxation in obstetrics and strong suggestion, mesmerism or hypnotism.'

One hundred years after the work of his compatriot Braid, Read still considered hypnosis as a 'mysterious power'.* In fact, the way in which Read reports the results of relaxation in certain of his better educated patients makes it difficult for the reader to escape the conclusion that they were related to hypnotic states. 'I have now had many such cases, and some of them have appeared to be lying in a trance from the beginning of their labour until the end. It is not that they were in a trance, but their relaxation was so complete that they became almost oblivious to the fact of parturition, and at the end of the first stage relaxation during the contractions of the so-called pain-period of labour enabled them to pass through it without discomfort. They then automatically brought into play the muscles of expulsion; they continued to lie in a completely relaxed state between the contractions, but woke up in a muscularly active condition to the full participation in expulsive effort. As soon as a contraction had worn off, these women again sank into an amnesic, almost anaesthetic state, for there is no doubt that general relaxation intensifies that amnesic condition during the second stage of labour of which I have so frequently spoken'.

American writers such as KROGER [284] and MANDY et al. [346] have not failed to notice this. It is very difficult not to reconcile Read's description with those of older authors when describing women who were being delivered under somnambulism. Read appears to ignore the fact that hypnosis is not a synonym for true sleep, and that a deep hypnotic state can be accompanied by conversation. Thus Read in fact sometimes practised hypnosis without knowing it.†

3. APPLICATIONS

A physiotherapist, Heardman, in Great Britain, has been largely responsible for propagating Read's method in England and the United States, and thereby insisting on the physiotherapeutic

*In the 1953 edition of *Childbirth without Fear*, Read, answering Kroger, expresses a less definite opinion about hypnosis.

†The much debated problem which arises here—namely the relationship between hypnosis and the educational methods (Natural Childbirth, Psychoprophylactic Method) will be taken up again later.

aspects of the method. She began a course of preparation for childbirth at University College Hospital in London, in the Unit directed by Professor NIXON. These courses were enlarged, and by 1951 Professor NIXON could write that they constituted the most important part of the prenatal care which was given at University College Hospital [396]. After having carried out the method for five years, in 1953 NIXON presented a statistical analysis bearing on the results in 600 cases, using an equal number of controls (a statistical expert also studied the figures). Nixon considered that the results showed little difference in the mechanical aspects of labour (its duration, lacerations, etc.) between women who had undergone training and those who had not, but emotionally the mothers who followed the course of preparation presented less tension and fear [397]. RANSOM [450], working under Professor Nixon in London, introduces the obstetrical team to the patient during her preparation. She recommends the presence of the husband during the childbirth. She points out that physical exercise can alter the body structurally very little unless it has been carried out from an early age but that physical education during pregnancy can play an important part in the psychological preparation.

ROBERTS et al. [469], of London, studied 1000 patients between 1949 and 1952 using a control group of 3000 patients. They found that prenatal preparation did not make labour shorter or easier, nor was it able to diminish the number of perineal tears. They believe however that it would be a serious error only to consider numerical factors, because it appears that there is no way of measuring the tranquility and feeling of security which occurs in these mothers as a result of prenatal preparation. 'They experience comfort and satisfaction in knowing what happens during labour and in the knowledge that they can do a lot to help themselves. The mother should not be made to think she has failed in her mission if some sedative has had to be given to help her . . . too enthusiastic teachers of antenatal exercises and relaxation have a tendency to regard any sedation as a confession of failure. It is important that we should adapt our methods . . . to the needs of the mother and not vice versa'.

SOLDENHOF [508], in Scotland, analysed the case records of 1000 prepared by a physiotherapist according to Read's method.

The deliveries took place between 1948 and 1954 in a hospital where, over the same period, there were 13,000 deliveries. He evaluated the results with regard to the administration of drugs. For 25 per cent no drugs were necessary and the results were excellent; in 50 per cent 100 mg of pethidine were needed and the results were good; in 20 per cent the dose was higher than 100 mg and the results were fairly good; the rest were failures. Soldenhof attached great importance to the element of suggestion: the secret undoubtedly lies in the patient being well 'indoctrinated with plenty of suggestion. In the future this might be carried a step further, to the use of hypnosis in obstetrics'. He believes that the continual presence of the doctor or the midwife near the woman in labour is of the first importance. Unhappily it is difficult to do this in hospital. The solution to the problem of obstetrical analgesia lies in 'a happy combination of relaxation and analgesics'.

Following the work of Helen Heardman, British physiotherapists showed great interest in the new method. One of them, EBNER [141], underlined the importance of the psychosomatic outlook in this method, pointing out the close interreaction of physical and mental phenomena in all branches of medicine. The aim of the method is to prepare the mother to carry out a natural physiological function, and by this means to develop in her the confidence in her ability to do so. Another English physiotherapist, MADDERS [343], recognizes the psychotherapeutic aspects of natural childbirth and, above all, emphasizes group psychotherapy. To take part in a group is an essential part of the therapy. Individual instruction, however far one takes it, can never supply the stimulus and the emulation that one finds in a group of mothers forming a single whole. In learning physical exercises to produce muscular relaxation, the woman acquires a weapon to fight her tension and her anxiety. The general muscular relaxation which ought to produce mental tranquillity will be of much more use to those in whom it is necessary for the work of labour. MONTGOMERY [373], a physiotherapist at Bristol Maternity Hospital, pleads for an 'active' conception of childbirth, and recommends the integration of physiotherapists into a harmonious obstetrical team.

BURNETT [68], of the West Middlesex Hospital, has attempted to study the influence of prenatal exercises on childbirth. Out of a yearly total of 2675 deliveries 287 women were studied. They had carried out exercises under the direction of a physiotherapist (and midwife) following the technique of Heardman, Read's disciple. At the same time they were given psychological instruction aiming at the suppression of fear, and the fostering of confidence. Burnett used the length of labour and the number of obstetrical complications as criteria by which to evaluate the results. He believes that pain cannot, in fact, be estimated by an objective measure. He found that 'Despite much painstaking and persevering work on the part of doctors, midwives and physiotherapists, antenatal relaxation and exercises have no influence on the length and character of labour'. Nevertheless, he allows that these exercises can have a useful postnatal effect, for instance, on lactation and the capacity of the woman 'to cope with her household duties'. But he sees this as 'the result of psychological preparation mediated through the exercises'.

For all that he is sceptical about psychotherapy, justifying his attitude by referring to the fact that midwives and doctors undergoing the method themselves have difficult childbirths. How could psychotherapy be successful with ordinary women when it may be a failure in well-informed women? In addition, he states that psychiatrists have no more confidence in the psychotherapeutic element, and he quotes CRAMOND [107] who found that women showing the least anxiety had difficult childbirths, and that 'fear, emotion and anxiety play no part from the practical, obstetrical point of view'.

The important thing, Burnett maintains, is the close co-operation between the patient and the midwife who cares for her throughout pregnancy and labour. This ought to be marked by confidence and affection. He adds that the relationship of the physiotherapist with the group cannot in any case usurp the interpersonal relationship between the midwife and patient. These views call for some comment.

Burnett has not succeeded in assessing the value of prenatal exercises for the very good reason that it is impossible to measure their influence outside the framework of a relationship. As we have seen, the psychotherapeutic factor is essential in all methods. Burnett at first seems to agree with this when he insists on the importance of the relationship between patient and midwife. But it is difficult to understand why, whilst admitting this, he denies the importance of psychotherapy. Is it that psychotherapy, for him, consists in education? This seems to be his opinion when he considers the difference between ordinary pregnant women and pregnant midwives or doctors. With regard to the anxiety, it is sometimes possible for women who show little anxiety to have difficult births. But there is another type of anxiety which shows no apparent sign of its presence, but influences childbirth at a much deeper level. GOODRICH [194], a follower of Read's method, recognized this type of anxiety, and saw in it the cause for many of the failures with the method. But he has also stated that women showing overt anxiety during their pregnancy may sometimes have easier births than others who do not show it, which proves that overt, expressed anxiety is not all. (Incidentally, this deep, concealed anxiety will be difficult to uncover, cf. p. 198). Cramond also stated, after studying 50 women presenting uterine dysfunction during labour, that they were more neurotic than a control group. It means that they had more anxiety but in a form which was not overtly manifest.

Another astonishing fact is that Burnett recognizes only an individual psychotherapeutic relationship—rejecting a group relationship. It seems then that Burnett takes up a very guarded view of the method he was using. Under these conditions it is not remarkable that the number of women taking part were so few; he writes 'in spite of persuasion, only 20 per cent of primiparae and three per cent of multiparae agreed to follow the preparation'. All of which confirms the importance of an enthusiastic approach by the doctor in winning recruits for the preparation, as well as its importance on the results. Deprived of its emotional context and reduced to a mechanical preparation, the method is useless.

SERVICE [505], a physiotherapist from New Zealand, also described her own practice of natural childbirth in that country.

STERNWEILER [511] carries out preparation for Natural Childbirth in Cape Town, South Africa.

HALL [216], The Honorary Obstetrician at the King Edward Memorial Hospital at Perth in Australia, practises Natural Childbirth. He considers it is a method to which the practitioner ought not to be opposed, as 'He will be the loser, because Natural

Childbirth patients are usually the most intelligent and grateful patients in one's practice'.

He believes that the presence of someone in whom the woman has great confidence, associated with lumbar massage, 'will do more to relieve the pain of labour than all the drugs at our command'.

Natural Childbirth for him only represents a stage, to be followed by another where less harmful medicaments may be used.

In the United States, SAWYER [490] pioneered the English method and published his first paper in 1946.

In January 1947, Read made a lecture tour in America on the invitation of the Maternity Centre Association [545]. This organization, which is under the direction of Hazel Corbin, has been concerned for the last twenty years or so with training obstetric nurses.* HAZEL CORBIN considers that they are the only persons qualified to adapt the accepted medical hospital and nursing routines to the mother's needs [93]. The aim of this association is to promote research, and grants have been given to medical and nursing personnel of obstetric units, enabling them to study the technique of Natural Childbirth.

Benefiting by this help, Herbert Thoms, Professor of Obstetrics and Gynaecology at Yale University started the method about 1947 in collaboration with Goodrich and others. He drew on the techniques of Read, Heardman and Jacobson. In 1950 three publications appeared, *Training for Childbirth*, by THOMS, *Understanding Natural Childbirth*, by THOMS et al. and *Natural Childbirth* by GOODRICH. In 1954 GELB recounted her experience of her own labour in a book designed for a large public, *The ABC of Natural Childbirth*. About 1948 THOMS published his first paper with Goodrich reporting on 156 pregnancies [193]. In 1949 the same writers reported a study of 546 cases [529]. In 1951 THOMS published with WYATT his results in 1000 cases [534]. In 1954 THOMS and KARLOVSKY reported their results in 2000 women delivered according to their method between January 1949 and April 1952 [532]. In addition to the usual prenatal preparation and assistance during delivery, which is the keystone of the method, Thoms introduced prenatal (paediatric) consul-

*They are midwives with training as nurses. The midwife, as understood in Europe, has no corresponding partner in the U.S.A.

tations for the mothers as well as 'rooming-in' for the mother and child, if the mother so desired. With regard to the use of drug analgesia, he left this to the woman herself to decide. From a theoretical point of view, Thoms did not accept all Read's postulates; thus he did not share the opinion that the fear of labour is a product of civilization. He pointed out that certain ethnological studies had shown that this fear existed in primitive societies. The expression 'Natural Childbirth' did not seem to him appropriate. About 1949 he came under the influence of psychoanalytically oriented writings, chiefly those of Helene Deutsch, which he mentioned in his introduction to *Training for Childbirth*. He quotes from her as follows: 'it is valuable therefore to gain an insight into the psychologic reactions of a woman who is delivered spontaneously, that is, into the greatest of all female pleasure-pains and its accompanying psychologically determined disturbances, before modern technic has deprived psychiatrists of the possibility of doing so'. Thoms has therefore collaborated with psychiatrists, obstetricians and pediatricians, who have brought a psychodynamic orientation to this problem of psychological analgesia.

These research workers have studied above all the factor of amnesia in delivery, and its relationships with pain, anxiety and the conflictual situations of women, FRIEDMAN *et al*. [173]. Whilst recognizing the importance of the experience which a woman lives through in a spontaneous delivery, Thoms does not insist too much upon this. In practice he uses drug analgesia 'when the woman demands it'. In certain cases he explains to the woman the advantage of operative assistance the indications for which remain just the same as before the application of the method. It is well known that in the U.S.A. the indications for this are very numerous [531]. At a psychotherapeutic level, whilst admitting the importance of emotional factors in the parturient woman and of the doctor-patient relationship, THOMS writes 'any idea that hypnosis or suggestion-therapy are factors should be dispelled' [530].

A word as to the results; of 2000 women certain of them (the percentage is not indicated) had followed the complete preparation, others had only partially been prepared, others did not even benefit from the method except in an extempore way. There were 703 primiparae and 1297 multiparae. Of the deliveries 34·2 per cent (660) were carried out without any drug; 62·0 per cent (1195) with pethidine (125 mg); 29·1 per cent (562) had no narcosis at the phase of expulsion; in 66·1 per cent (1275) the anaesthesia was limited to the intermittent inhalation of trilene or of nitrous oxide. One hundred and twenty-three women had a general anaesthetic, of whom 73 were submitted to Caesarian section. One hundred and sixty-six underwent a forceps delivery. THOMS lists the following as advantages of the method: a diminution in the number of babies needing resuscitation, a reduction in the length of labour, the number of obstetrical operations and of haemorrhages and, he adds, 'happier mothers, and parents better adapted to the start of family life' [531].

THOMS and BILLINGS [537] insist on the idea that 'the key to success in any childbirth programme is skilled and sympathetic attendance for the woman in active labour'. Another problem with which Thoms is concerned is that of the personnel preparing the woman. He comes out in favour of training more midwives. One obstetrician has insufficient time to give to the woman so as to provide moral support. Accordingly the midwife ought to play an important part in the pre-, peri- and postnatal periods, whilst still remaining under the control of the doctor.

BUXTON [70], Thoms' successor at Yale, is more guarded in his attitude toward prepared childbirth. He has now begun an objective study which in a few years will allow of an objective evaluation of this method of childbirth. For the time being, he confines himself to the recognition of certain subjective advantages: 'It has the definite psychologic advantage of occupying the patient's attention and making her feel, during labour, that she is efficiently contributing to the process'.

DAVIDSON [113], of New York, practises Read's method, but prefers the expression 'Educated Childbirth' to that of Natural Childbirth.

He defined 'Educated Childbirth' as 'the conduct of labour characterized by the education of the pregnant woman to endure and master her labour with a minimum of analgesia and anaesthesia'. The essential feature of the method is the active participation of the woman in her childbirth. He was led to Natural Childbirth after being impressed by the numerous women who wanted to have it, and on the other hand, by the fact that on drug is free from danger. He reviews the writings dealing with the ill-effects of drugs on the mother and child in obstetrics. There are some who even see a relationship between cerebral palsy and foetal anoxia during labour (DEAVER [115] and Faber). The psychological advantage which the mother derives from living through her childbirth is added to the lessened risk from drugs.

In a work published in 1953, DAVIDSON [114] laid stress on the psychosomatic aspects of the preparation, insisting on a permissive regime divested of all exaggerated discipline. If the woman does not put into effect the orders she is given she may get a detrimental psychological effect from it. He gives her drugs on demand. He does not contradict those who speak of the contractions as pains because he does not treat the parturient woman as a child. He has had experience of 122 cases. MILLER et al. [368] of Cedar Rapids, Iowa, have published results based on 450 cases; VAN AUKEN and TOMLINSON [546] of Troy, New York, have studied 200 cases. DE LEE and DUNCAN [120] practise Read's method in Chicago. De Lee is an obstetrician, Duncan a nurse with knowledge of the physiology, anatomy and psychology of pregnancy and labour. De Lee believes that it is legitimate to entrust the preparation to a competent nurse, as she can give more time than the busy obstetrician. Moreover he considers that pregnant women are more able to talk woman-to-woman on intimate matters*.

LAIRD and HOGAN [292] carried out a study between May 1951 and June 1953, under the auspices of the Presbyterian Hospital, the Maternity Centre Association and the New York Foundation on Natural Childbirth, at the Sloane Hospital, New York. Seven hundred and forty-two unselected women were asked to follow the courses of preparation for childbirth; 515 showed interest, but only 283 undertook the course. The group was reinforced by 249 women who themselves asked to take part. They came from both private and hospital patients. Amongst the parturients, some wanted to be left in peace, others wanted encouragement; some wanted to see the birth, others preferred to be asleep. Again some wanted to see the child soon after the birth, others were too tired to make the effort. It was also noted that the woman's

*Hellman has an opposite view. He thinks that the pregnant woman is more confident with a male doctor.

behaviour was assessed differently by the obstetrician and the patient, as shown by the following table based on 230 deliveries:

	Mothers	Obstetricians
Successful	142	150
Reasonably successful	46	24
Fairly successful	32	24
Unsuccessful	10	27

A reduction of two hours in the duration of labour was recorded in primiparae, and there was a diminution in the use of anaesthetics and analgesiants for the whole group. This was more marked in those women who had opted for the method on their own initiative.

At several places in the U.S.A. associations have been founded to spread the ideas of Natural Childbirth. MURPHY [377], for instance, reports the existence of such an association in Milwaukee, Wisconsin; a panel of nurses attend to the preparation of the future mothers and even takes them to the hospital in order to give them moral support during the coming labour.

ROGERS [474], of Washington, draws attention to the dangers which may occur with Read's method for patients with major personality problems. He does not deny the usefulness of the method, provided that it is applied judiciously. But he has found that there is a group of neurotic or psychotic women who are obsessed with the idea of Natural Childbirth. He reports nine cases where the women developed psychotic reactions after childbirth conducted by Read's method, which they themselves had requested. However, in our opinion, it would seem difficult to impute these disturbances to the preparation; there is nothing which prevents us assuming that they could have been produced quite apart from the preparation. Nonetheless it is desirable that such cases should be recognized and receive appropriate care. Hence the importance of a close collaboration between obstetricians and psychiatrists in the same team, so that the preparation can also be used for the recognition of psychiatric disturbances in the pregnant woman.

In Canada, TUPPER [544] of Halifax used the method between 1950–54, and named it 'Conditioning for Childbirth'. His experience comprises 1200 cases. At the outset he declared that he was sceptical chiefly of all that concerned analgesia. 'After four years' experience we are still sceptical of some of the claims made for it but those of us who have given it a fair trial are now convinced that it can become a very valuable factor in solving the problems of childbirth'. The criteria of the worth of the method for this writer are as follows: excellent results, corresponding to deliveries conducted without any sedative or using local anaesthesia for passage of the head; very good results for those cases where sedatives have been employed; good for those where trilene had to be administered; 'helped' for those in whom delivery necessitated a general anaesthetic. He classes as failures those women who declare that they do not want to undergo the method again for their future deliveries. His results are shown in the following table:

	Primiparae per cent	Multiparae per cent
Excellent	19·7	46·5
Very good	22·6	10·7
Good	27·7	17·8
Helped	22·0	17·8
Failures	8·0	7·2

Tupper considers the advantages of the method for the child. There is no longer the problem of the resuscitation of the newborn 'Natural Childbirth babies are better babies. They breathe and cry more spontaneously, are less irritable, are happier. . . . '. 'The reduction in the number of times forceps are needed varies from 30 per cent to 18 per cent and with the result that 'fewer babies are as tense and difficult as any type of forceps baby tends to be'. As to feeding, women who were prepared for childbirth seemed to have a greater sense of their duties towards the child, which results in a higher percentage of women ready to breastfeed. Sixty-five per cent of women fed their children as against 50 per cent in the controlled group. The psychological benefits are very important to the woman, if one considers that 'for the great majority of married women, having a baby is the most important thing that they do—the one thing they can do that we men cannot do—our domination of their pregnancy and delivery robs them of a considerable amount of the psychological satisfaction they might derive from the process'. Tupper's exercises are considerably simplified and consist principally of three: (1) deep inspiration and expiration in the first phase of delivery; (2) panting respirations during the last half hour before complete dilatation, when the contractions are very painful; and (3) learning how to make the expulsive efforts. Relaxation is preferred not only during contractions, but also during the intervals between them. PORTNUFF [432], of Montreal, has also studied 222 pregnant women in his practice prepared for childbirth by Read's method.

To return to Europe, in the Netherlands KLOOSTERMAN [272] and VAN EPS [148, 149] have practised Read's methods since 1949 at the Maternity Hospital of the School for Midwives in Amsterdam. Van Eps thinks that it is particularly interesting to verify this method in Holland where, in general, it is considered that the normal woman in good health ought not to have recourse to a narcotic to relieve the pain of normal childbirth. Van Eps has studied 335 cases prepared by Read's method. The already low number of disturbed parturients in Holland, was still further diminished thanks to this method.

In France MAYER [358], drawing inspiration from the work of Read and Thoms, has practised the method of Natural Childbirth since 1948. Since 1954 he added 'psychological education and practice in child-rearing before and after childbirth' [353]. Moreover, he became interested in the psychological problems of pregnant women and his psychiatric assistants have dealt with these problems in group psychotherapy. From the theoretical point of view, Mayer, whilst maintaining the priority of Read's method in point of time, has recognized that Russian physiologists, inspired by Pavlovian concepts, have provided sound physiological, psychological and methodological criteria for the conceptions which Read originally put forward [355]. In his practice, Mayer uses no one technique, drawing from Read, as well as borrowing elements from Velvovski.* Mayer has studied, since 1950, 2760 cases, contrasting them with an equal number of traditional deliveries. It is interesting to note that the proportion of patients demanding succour from the method have changed from 7 per cent in 1949 to 55 per cent in 1956 [356]. RAIMBAULT [447], the psychosomatic assistant of Mayer, has written a thesis in which she has analysed 800 case records. With regard to the analgesia itself the factors leading to success lie in the persistence in following the

*A general tendency can be seen in France and in other European countries not to separate these two closely related techniques. See discussion in Chapter 11.

courses of anatomy and the conferences with the psychiatrists, rather than in persistence with physical training. Factors accounting for failure include pathological pregnancies and incomplete preparation. From the obstetrical point of view, if one compares natural deliveries and classical deliveries, it is found that in the first group a larger number of spontaneous deliveries occur; that is to say, deliveries without any oxytoxic drug or sedative being used. The duration of labour is appreciably diminished, and the percentage of 'immediate cries' is higher amongst children who are born by means of Natural Childbirth. Raimbault has also obtained very good results with difficult women and those likely to be failures by practising group psychotherapy with them.

LEPAGE and LANGEVIN-DROGUET [321] of Paris have practised Read's method since 1949, after reading Read's book and seeing what was being done in London and Stockholm. They consider that 'pain is one of the principal characteristics of uterine contractions in labour, it is physiological and no theory can change that'. The aim of the method is 'to instil confidence into the woman, to enable her to go through labour without fear and without feeling any anxiety or apprehension'. They included massage in their technique, and this takes place during the last ten minutes of the usual training sessions. LANGEVIN-DROGUET [308] describes them as follows. 'Massage of the limbs and of the back, not because it has itself any profound effect, but at the beginning of each session it allows for a transition from the outer world, a putting at ease, and above all it gives the physiotherapist contact with the woman, so that she can deal with what is upsetting her patient, and allow her to talk freely of her pregnancy and of her delivery.' LEPAGE and LANGEVIN-DROGUET consider that 'the results, which are difficult to account for, are achieved chiefly by the change in the atmosphere in the labour wards, where silence and calm now reign' [321]. As an example they studied the character of the labours in forty primiparae who had been prepared, and of forty who had not been prepared. The duration of labour was the same, but there were less forceps applications, and less perineal tears amongst the women who had been prepared. In 1957 [322] they reported a statistical analysis begun in 1955 by the National Institute of Hygiene. There were 535 cases; results were excellent in 32·5 per cent, very good in 26·6 per cent, fair in 20·0 per cent, and failures in 20·9 per cent. They demonstrated a significant difference with regard to the child's first cry; delayed by less than 5 minutes, 2·9 per cent instead of 15 per cent; delayed by more than 5 minutes, 1·2 per cent instead of 6 per cent. HARLIN [219], a physiotherapist, and a former associate of Lepage, published in 1951 a brochure for the general public entitled *Prepare Yourself for a Happy Maternity*.

In Lyon, NOTTER [401], after having seen the method practised at University College Hospital in London in 1952, read a paper at the Society of Obstetrics and of Gynaecology at Lyon. He succinctly described the practice of the method. A year later, before the same society, Notter gave a brief appreciation of Read's method [402]. He felt that relaxation was an important part of the method, and that it facilitated dilatation. He believed that the rest cures practised in certain tuberculosis sanatoria involved some degree of relaxation, and this might explain why these patients delivered themselves more easily than others. Working with Bansillon at the Maternity Hospital of the Hotel Dieu in Lyon between 1948 and 1953, of a total of 11,982 deliveries there were 81 amongst tuberculous patients; Notter was able to confirm that these deliveries were quicker and less painful than the others. All the parturient women came from sanatoria where they had been submitted to rest cures isolated from their familial tenvironment [30].

NOTTER and EGRON [403], in 1956 analysed 253 births amongst patients with pulmonary tuberculosis, carried out in two maternity units in Lyon. There was a grand total of 27,000 deliveries in these two units between 1950 and 1954. The women with tuberculosis had easier and shorter labours (for primiparae 10 hours and for multiparae 6 hours). These women had not been prepared, but the writers believed that they had undergone a spontaneous preparation; the physical side had been dealt with by the rest cure, itself very similar to relaxation. The psychological effect had been brought about by the isolation from the home environment and by the optimistic outlook in the hospital. Moreover, a new conditioning had been created in the cortex through 'the diversion of the preoccupation with childbirth toward the tuberculosis'.*

*The problem of easier childbirth in tuberculous patients seems to deserve a more detailed study. It appears that these writers consider

In 1954 BANSILLON and NOTTER [29] delivered thirty primiparae in a private clinic. They prefer to speak of childbirth without fear, rather than of childbirth without pain. Of the women 50 per cent were able to go through their expulsive phase in complete calm, and in only 20 per cent of cases was pain diminished but not entirely suppressed. Of the patients 50 per cent claimed an anaesthetic at the end of dilatation. PIGEAUD [417] considers that the Russian obstetricians have 'taken up Read's studies, and whilst developing them, have given a physiological basis on Pavlovian lines to the methods of preparation'. It is naïve to speak of childbirth without pain, because all childbirth is painful, and he therefore proposes the name of 'childbirth with diminished pain'. In 1956 PIGEAUD and NOTTER [418] named their technique 'psychophysiotherapeutic prophylactic preparation for childbirth'. At this time, after 18 months' experience they had dealt with several hundreds of cases. Only primiparae were considered in assessing their results; satisfactory results rose to 85 per cent. They believed that psychophysiotherapeutic prophylactic preparation was of interest 'because these methods were a useful complement, and in practice must be associated with other methods of relieving pain'.

PIGEAUD et al. [419] report their results in 316 primiparae. These women had carried out three to six training sessions, the number of sessions having no effect on the results. In general the

---

relaxation as a purely physical factor and underestimate its psychotherapeutic importance. The state of relaxation is propitious for both auto- and heterosuggestion (taken in its best sense). Moreover, the solicitude of the doctor, as of the nursing personnel, is usually increased when the pregnant woman has some physical handicap. We have ourselves observed two women, one of whom, suffering from coxalgia, had had her first pregnancy terminated by miscarriage, and the other was a primipara with a contracted pelvis. The first had been discarded from the group undergoing normal preparation because of her anxiety. The second had not been prepared and found herself anxious at the prospect of a Caesarian section. Both of them had been hospitalized for several days before the childbirth and both were given a rapid preparation by hypnoid relaxation, to which they responded well. The anxiety disappeared and the two women went through labour in a complete waking state, in a most painless and rapid manner. Both of them received particular attention from us, as well as from the whole of the personnel.

authors recommend six sessions; in those cases where the woman has carried out no preparation psychophysiotherapeutic training should be attempted when she arrives in the maternity clinic. They mention a reduction in the number of forcep applications; only 28 out of 316 who had been prepared, instead of 53 in the control group. On the other hand they report five cases out of 288 women where the baby needed resuscitation, as against one single case in the control group.

NOTTER [404], in 1957 analysed 1243 patients who had been prepared by the psychophysiotherapeutic method, to which spirometry had been added (the spirometer is a simple gasometric device). In addition to the physical effect of oxygenation, he stresses the psychological action of the respiratory rhythm. 'A good respiratory rhythm maintains the morale of the victor in an athletic competition'. The technique consists in 15–20 minute group sessions. They 'breathe in time and carry out their respiratory manoeuvres together under the direction of the midwife or of the physiotherapist'. The sight of the graduated cylinder marking the women's efforts tells them whether their exercise is being successful; those who best succeeded in this exercise obtained the better deliveries. Notter believes that this method has many advantages. Spirometric exercises produce a good oxygenation, as well as a general effect on relaxation and constitute a cortical activity. It produces, moreover, a competitive spirit amongst the women and increases contact between them and the staff.

In Switzerland, VON RUTTE [482], of Berne, in 1951 reviewed the British method. He laid stress chiefly on the physiological rather than the psychological aspects of the method. Of primary importance were the respiratory exercises and relaxation; then came 'muscular training'. His views had been formed at the Karolinska Hospital in Stockholm. As distinct from Read, von Rutte did not obtain analgesia by this prenatal preparation. He was able to obtain some slight diminution in the use of chemical anaesthetics; about half of the women needed nitrous oxide plus dolantin. About a quarter of the patients received only dolantin, and a quarter were delivered without any anaesthetic. The amount of anaesthetic was less in the women who had been prepared than in the other patients; he also noticed more rapid recovery from childbirth.

Von Rust [480] of Zurich treated 600 women in a four-year period using Read's method; he was able to analyse his results in 101 of them. Amongst other advantages he noted an appreciable reduction in the length of labour, by five hours in primiparae, and three hours in the multiparae. In 1956 [481] Von Rust tried to quantify the different elements of the method. He believes that the didactic factor plays a part in 50–60 per cent of the method, respiratory exercises and relaxation in 30–35 per cent of the method and physical exercises in 5–20 per cent. This latter should not be neglected because it can increase the strength of the whole relationship.

Merz [361] of the Gynaecological Clinic at Basle, also believes that it is important not to neglect physical exercises. He sees no difference between the Russian and English methods. His experience is related to 152 women in his hospital practice and 104 from his private practice. Sauter [489], of Zurich, considers that the theoretical bases of the British and Russian methods are identical. He wonders whether, physiologically, uterine contractions are painful; after all, he says, there are no physiological functions accompanied by pain. He believes that pain is the result of 'a dyskinesia of a functional disorder'. Mieville [367], of Chexbres, for the last two years at the hospital in Lavaux has used an eclectic method based on the works of Read, Velvovski, Platonov, Nicolaiev, Lamaze and on those of the physiotherapeutic schools in Germany (Kohlrausch, Terrich-Schultz), in Switzerland (Liechti), in England (Morris-Heardman), and in America (Jacobson). The phrase Natural Childbirth seems more reasonable and less open to criticism than that of Painless Childbirth.

In Germany Lukas [337] practised Read's method at Giessen; Hellmann [226], of Hamburg, has practised Read's method since 1949. He became interested in the psychological aspects of obstetrics after being influenced by the theories of 'organismic' psychotherapy put forward by J. H. Schultz. He alludes to the 'intra-uterine education of the child' and to the influence of the state of the mother's mind on the foetus. Thus by working on the mother he would thereby carry out a foetal psychotherapy. He insists on the importance of living through the experience of childbirth, saying that drug-induced anaesthesia deprives the woman of the 'orgasm of birth'. In his practice Hellmann adds to Read's methods the most simple exercises of the Autogenous Training.* He also uses light hypnosis to reinforce Read's method [227].

LOHMER [333], of Munich, in 1955 reported 200 cases prepared by this method. He obtained a diminution of the pain and a mean reduction in labour of four hours for primiparae and five hours for multiparae. He found that the mean duration of labour was 13 hours, calculating this on a method used by Schildbach in 20,000 deliveries. SCHIRMACHER [493] describes a preparation for childbirth, based on positive persuasion and a psychological and physical training. He frequently employed spasmolytics.

MARTIUS [349], of the Obstetrical University Clinic in Munich (1956), also interested himself in Read's methods. For him childbirth is a physiological phenomenon, but different from other such phenomena because of the danger of haemorrhage, of tears, etc. Pain here acts as a warning signal. He is in favour of the midwife taking a large part in the preparation, believing, as he does, that the obstetrician has not always enough time. To avoid deceptions it is important not to promise a painless childbirth. In Austria SCHMIEDECK [494], at the Semmelweiss Clinic in Vienna in 1953, reopened the problem of obstetrical analgesia. After describing drug analgesia, he mentions that hypnosis is useful in certain cases, but cannot be used in general. He then mentions a technique of analgesia practised in the United States by the use of music and of colours. Musical airs and certain colours play a part in the emotional state of the parturient women in the same way as an analgesic. Schmiedeck himself practises Read's method and reports fifty cases delivered with this method. Ninety per cent of these deliveries were made without any medication. Forceps were not necessary but in order to evaluate the method without recourse to the element of suggestion, the doctor was absent during the delivery.†

In Italy, DELLEPIANE of Turin began by using Read's method. With his collaborators, Davitti, Bocci, Chiudano, Pinoli and

*He does not use a true combination of Read's method and of Autogenous Training, as does PRILL [435], another German worker (cf.p. 85).

†The absence of the accoucheur does not do away with the element of suggestion, which is already operative during the training sessions. Amongst others Read himself has drawn attention to the beneficial effect of suggestion.

Terzi, he has developed a method, adapted for Italian women, which draws inspiration from both Russian and English techniques [123, 124, 48, 49].

Bocci and Davitti [50] have studied the psychological reactions of women with prolonged pregnancies. They present a statistical analysis of 700 women who had been prepared between February 1955 and February 1957. A control group was also used consisting of 4046 women. In the first group there were 8·2 per cent of prolonged pregnancies as against 14 per cent in the second group. They believe that prolonged pregnancy influences the behaviour of the woman during labour, making it not so good. On this account it is necessary to warn women during preparation of the possibility of a prolonged pregnancy, and to prepare them for this.

Chiaudano and Pinoli [89] insist on the use of films and cartoons in preparation. They believe 'the teaching film is a modern means of rational education in the conditioning of the pregnant woman'. Terzi [525] studied *The Importance of Psychomotor Relationships in Natural Childbirth.*

In Spain, Ferreira Gomez [160] practised a combined method derived from both Read and Velvovski. In Portugal Nogueira [399] has drawn attention to Read's method as practised in the service of M. Mayer in Paris.

The British method has also been practised for several years in the Scandinavian countries, and is beginning to be used in South America.

4. AMERICAN CRITICISMS

The criticisms of Read's method have been made by the adherents of the hypnosuggestive method (Kroger, Abramson and Heron), by followers of drug-produced analgesia (Mandy *et al.* [346]), and by Jacobson on the problem of relaxation. All groups, whilst expressing reserve with regard to the scientific value of Read's conception agree in recognizing his human qualities and his merits as a pioneer in the introduction of a psychosomatic point of view to obstetrics. A point of view, moreover, which has taken into account the emotional needs of the woman. After criticizing the absence of a physiological basis for the method, and the name Natural Childbirth, Kroger [284] puts forward his chief argument against Read, namely that the main factor in his method is hypnosis. If the patients were not in a deep hypnotic state, then they were in a state of 'waking hypnosis', during which all hypnotic phenomena can be obtained without the necessity of sleep. (This is a technique elaborated by Wells, inspired by Bernheim's description of 'suggestion á l état de veille'.) This latter state implies no loss of consciousness. On the other hand Kroger reproaches Read for likening hypnosis to natural sleep, which it is not. He considers with Brenman and Gill that 'even deeply hypnotized persons are fully conscious, and may be completely aware of all sensations, as in the so-called waking state' [284]. MANDY et al. [347] also criticized Read for having taken too superficial a view of fear. Anxiety during pregnancy is not the result of a simple feeling of fear of childbirth, it has deeper roots in the personality and is related to psychosexual maturity, relationships with parents, brothers, and sisters, friends, etc. Other fears are bound up with economic and social problems, and the woman can equally well be afraid of aesthetic misfortunes. The pain of childbirth is natural and it can be intensified by unconscious emotional conflicts. These latter are not accessible to the peripheral approach which this method employs. The authors note that Goodrich himself, one of the chief proponents of the method, thinks that it may apply only to superficial conscious strata, and that women who have profound anxiety constitute the failures. Mandy and his co-workers further consider that hypnosis and relaxation are phenomena which are in a reciprocal relationship. Hypnosis is a continuum which runs from simple relaxation right up to somnambulism. The method of induction of a light trance is almost the same as that of the technique of relaxation. A determining factor in both is the need of the subject to enter into an interpersonal relationship with the therapist and to feel confidence in him and in his method. From the psychotherapeutic point of view, they believe that Read's method does not produce a maturation of the woman but 'encourages her dependence upon an important authoritative figure, supported by formal, complex and ritualistic routines' [347]. Mandy, using a technique of simple relaxation, was able to obtain an anaesthesia deep enough to carry out a Caesarian section on a woman suffering from a severe toxaemia in whom any pharmacological anaesthesia was contraindicated. With regard to the instruction of the patient, Mandy and his co-workers considered that to a certain extent they could produce a more rational approach to pregnancy and childbirth, but it was also possible for them to increase anxiety. As for the exercises, their use in producing an analgesia is difficult to measure. RODWAY [472] compared 340 pregnant women who carried out exercises, and an equal group who did not; she found no difference between the two groups as far as the pain of childbirth was concerned. The principal advantages of preparation consist in the personal attention which is given to the patient and the feeling of belonging to a group and being able to participate in a situation where a positive group feeling can occur.

With regard to the analgesia, these authors report the findings of JAVERT and HARDY [249] who measured the intensity of pain with an instrument they called the dolorimeter.* Javert and Hardy found that preparation by Read's method had no influence on the intensity of the pain. At the expulsive phase the reading was 10·5 dol which corresponds to a second degree burn. Nevertheless preparation produced a pattern of reaction comparable to that obtained with moderate doses of heroin, morphine or penthidine. Mandy *et al.* prefer pharmacological anaesthesia and do not believe, as Read does, that the waking state is emotionally necessary to those parturient women who have a very painful labour. The memory which can remain may in future have a traumatizing effect. If the participation of the woman in childbirth is really felt to be necessary then spinal anaesthesia should be used. Finally, they consider that the method is a useful adjuvant, which supports the patient emotionally, and diminishes the drugs needed. But it should not be held that every woman can be delivered by this method without suffering. This attitude would bring other therapeutic methods into disrepute.

With regard to hypnosis, FREEDMAN *et al.* [173], members of the group working with Thoms have replied to Kroger and

*The dolorimeter of HARDY *et al.* [218] is an apparatus using radiant heat to measure the subjective experience of pain. The measurement is made by comparing the pain which is felt subjectively with the pain which is produced by the apparatus. The intensity of pain is expressed in terms of dols. The value of this method is controversial.

Mandy that they have not encountered much amnesia in the course of childbirth carried out by Read's method. Hypnosis and amnesia being to their mind inseparable, they therefore conclude that the method is not accompanied by hypnosis. This argument, however, is not very convincing because hypnosis does not necessarily involve an amnesia. The amnesia can be very superficial and fleeting.*

Another forgotten point is that analgesia does not always result immediately from hypnosis, but is sometimes due to a posthypnotic effect (this is the principle on which Kogerer's work is based). If the interpersonal relationship produced in the hypnotic state is considered capable of producing an analgesia, and if it is considered a psychotherapeutic relationship of a particularly concentrated degree, one can imagine that all doctor–patient relationships are capable of producing a certain analgesic effect. The question of whether hypnosis enters into Read's method seems ill-conceived. The analgesiant mechanism resulting from the doctor–patient relationship in the waking state uses the same affective pathways as analgesia produced in the hypnotic relationship.

But whilst borrowing the same affective pathways, this analgesic process can take place at multiple levels of integration. Thus there is a difference between the action of the hypnosuggestive methods and the educational methods although the borderline is not definite. As the older experiences of somnambulistic analgesia show, even in this form of analgesia, the patterns adopted by the parturient women are different. In the educational methods, owing to the intervention of other elements such as information, learning, etc., the analgesia can also operate at other levels, but the experimental basis is not so obvious. To contend, as do Kroger and Mandy, that Read's technique is purely hypnotic would be to oversimplify the problem.†

*This superficial and fleeting character of hypnotic amnesia was shown by Bernheim. Freud records that Bernheim had shown him how one could easily bring back forgotten memories of what had happened during hypnosis. It was this that led Freud, without recourse to hypnosis, 'to bring back into consciousness forgotten facts and relationships' [177].

†VELVOVSKI [556] is in agreement with the American writers in considering that Read's method includes some hypnotic factors. It is therefore amusing to observe how these different writers reproach each

Edmund Jacobson of Chicago, the author of *Progressive Relaxation*, has been highly praised by followers of Read's method, but Jacobson himself, as we have already noted, has declared that his technique has been ill-understood and incorrectly applied. He particularly castigates the idea of 'relaxation exercises' which are found in many of the writings propagating Read's method. He criticizes these exercises for having been conceived in a 'positive' manner, that is to say, of being made up of a movement of contraction followed by the opposite movement of relaxation. For him his method ought always to be a negative process, a 'not doing' which cannot be brought about by means of exercises or of contractions which are 'positive'. Having noticed what happened when he contracts his muscles, the subject is invited to remain no longer in this attitude, but to let his muscles go, as Jacobson

---

other as carrying out hypnosis. Read, as we have seen, vigorously denies the allegation. Velvovski, whilst giving due credit to hypnosis in the genesis of his Psychoprophylactic Method, and whilst recognizing its great usefulness, excludes it from the practice of his method. Lamaze repudiates all relationship between hypnosis and the Psychoprophylactic Method. However, certain critics have maintained that there is a relationship, and de Watteville, the proponent of the Psychoprophylactic Method in Geneva, has had to vigorously reject this idea himself. He sees an essential difference between the two methods.

'In hypnotism the patient is in a cataleptic or lethargic state, whereas the parturient with psychoprophylactic preparation must be fully conscious and intellectually active. No dangerous emotional interdependence is established between the monitor and the patient, her personality is not disconnected and the subconscious mind is not affected as in hypnotism'. It can be seen that de Watteville in this respect finds himself much closer to Read than to Velvovski. Read, at least in the beginning, saw in hypnosis a dangerous procedure. Velvovski eliminates hypnosis because of the impracticability of its general use, and also for theoretical reasons. Hypnosis heals, whilst education prevents the pain. But he insists on the harmlessness of hypnosis both for the mother and the child.

It is certainly true that Read's description of some of his patients in childbirth recalls to mind the hypnotic state. In certain patients relaxation can induce hypnoid states, and these are very propitious to suggestibility, whether one interprets them in Pavlovian terms of inhibition or in psychoanalytic terms such as regression. Hypnoid states can also arise in patients on the analytic couch, but this does not mean that psychoanalysis is nothing more than suggestion. This problem will be discussed in Chapter 12.

says, to 'go negative'. The subject thus learns to feel his tensions, and to be able to disperse them any time that he may want to do so. Each muscular group in turns is taken in a predetermined order. The subject learns successively to relax the muscles of the arms, the legs, the abdomen, etc. To finish with, he takes notice of the tensions bound up in the muscles which mediate speech, 'counting from one to ten, imagining counting from one to ten and carrying out other acts of imaginary speech'. Jacobson has built an apparatus which he calls the 'electroneuromyometer' which measures the degree of tension of the muscles. By means of this apparatus he has demonstrated that relaxation exercises do not produce the muscular relaxation which he himself obtains by his own technique. He considers that his method is purely physiological and that the psychological aspects of the preparation for childbirth are completely useless. It is not necessary to (a) stimulate enthusiasm, (b) to cultivate faith or suggested states, and (c) to educate the pregnant woman in the mechanics of childbirth. These three measures can lead her to be overemotional and overreflective during labour. The teaching of relaxation is a purely technical affair, just as in teaching golf or swimming. He considers that interpersonal relationships are completely negligible and he eliminates all suggestion from his method, considering it to be prejudicial to the pregnant woman. Disagreeing with Read as he does in so many ways, Jacobson nevertheless inveighs with as much strength as Read against the idea that hypnosis or hypnoid states can have anything in common with relaxation. On the contrary he considers that hypnoid states imply tension, which he claims to have demonstrated by electromyographic means in his laboratory. By this method of relaxation alone, Jacobson intends to obtain a diminution in the reaction to the pain of childbirth, rather than a complete analgesia. But this method, when it is strictly followed, is very time-consuming, and up to the present has not been used in obstetrics on a large scale. In fact the author has reported on no more than a dozen cases between 1930 and 1954 [246].

5. READ'S METHOD COMBINED WITH THE AUTOGENOUS TRAINING OF J. H. SCHULTZ

The Autogenous Training or Konzentrative Selbstentspannung is derived, according to its author (SCHULTZ [497, 498]) 'from old-established and sure medical practices of hypnosis'. He considers that modern psychotherapy has neglected the body far too much. The technique of Autogenous Training is, the author believes, a psychotherapeutic technique, a technique which revalues the role of the body in the make-up of the patient's personality and in the process of his healing. For Schultz 'hypnosis is a state of repose resembling sleep',* it is produced by a purely psychological action, always successful in healthy people and more difficult amongst nervous patients. He lays much stress on 'the hypnotic state which, deprived of any external influence, is a state of internal concentration, producing a feeling of well-being, of repose and of calm'. Hypnosis, like sleep, constitutes a global state in which the body and the mind cannot be dissociated. In the hypnotic state, one sees bodily changes manifesting themselves by a heaviness which corresponds to muscular relaxation, and a warmth due to vascular dilatation. Cardiac, respiratory and other changes can also be obtained. In hypnosis as in sleep there is a 'disconnection' ('umschaltung'), a passage from a state of connection with the exterior world to a state of repose. The essential feature of this 'disconnection', in hypnosis as well as in sleep, is the relaxation which is found particularly in the muscles and in the blood vessels. This relaxation is not the concomitant of hypnosis but is its essential feature. The goal of Autogenous Training, which is a sort of fragmented autohypnosis, is to make the subject himself produce by means of exercises this state of relaxation, which is beneficial and curative. The exercises, six in number, are carried out in a certain order, so as to successively experience the weight of the limbs (muscular relaxation), the sensation of warmth in the limbs (vascular dilatation), modifications of the respiratory and cardiac rhythms, a feeling of warmth in the epigastric region, and a feeling of freshness in the forehead. Each exercise is repeated for about a fortnight. They consist of an active process of mental concentration on a bodily sensation. For instance the subject thinks, 'my arm is heavy' and a sensation of heaviness results which corresponds to a muscular relaxation. Schultz believes that by his method he can obtain psychotherapeutic results of appreciable worth, whilst reducing to a minimum the dependence of the subject on his doctor.

*Cf. [85].

The theoretical aspects of Schultz's method as well as certain of its therapeutic aspects have been studied in France by AJURIAGUERRA and BADARACCO [8], and by AJURIAGUERRA et al. [9]. A review of the therapeutic aspects of relaxation has been recently published by DEMANGEAT [125]. BURGER [65] has outlined the theoretical problems of Schultz's work. A collection of essays by the main representatives of the relaxation methods has been published (1958) under the auspices of the French Society of Psychosomatic Medicine [465].

The German accoucheur, PRILL [435] of Wurzbourg has combined Read's method with Schultz's technique. He believes that the important relaxation which is obtained by Autogenous Training augments the analgesic effect and results in greater successes than can be produced by the original method of Read; 125 cases were described. He considers there are two modes of action on the pregnant woman; the indirect or autogenous pathway, working through exercises, relaxation, Autogenous Training, etc. and the more direct or suggestive pathway by means of education, persuasion, suggestion or hypnosis. Although recognizing the efficacy and the innocuous quality of hypnosis and suggestion, he states that they cannot be applied generally, owing to the technical difficulties and the resistances which they provoke amongst certain doctors. In these circumstances, he considers that the method he has elaborated, which is based chiefly on an indirect or autogenous action, remains the most satisfactory method of producing a hypalgesia or an obstetrical analgesia. Prill's method comprises, as well as Autogenous Training, muscular and respiratory exercises and educational elements. Fourteen sessions are given, spread over the last three months of pregnancy, and three to five women make up a group. The three elements, Autogenous Training, exercise and education enter into each session.

(a) Physical Exercises

There are two kinds of exercise used by Prill: (a) relaxation exercises and (b) respiratory exercises.

(a) Muscular relaxation proceeds progressively, beginning with the muscles of the arm. At each session a different group of muscles is dealt with and the preceding groups are re-exercised.

At the fifth session, respiratory exercises are begun. Muscular relaxation should not be confused with the exercises used in Autogenous Training, which are independently carried out by the patient. Prill does not consider that muscular relaxation produces an analgesic effect.

(b) Prill attaches great importance to respiration, which has both a physical and a psychological influence. He tries to produce a good oxygenation, which is necessary for the severe work which the muscles will have to carry out during labour. Prill recommends a medium amplitude and frequency of respiration; he does not recommend too deep a respiration, in which there is an elimination of more carbon dioxide than is desirable, nor too superficial a respiration, which does not allow for an adequate supply of oxygen. He believes that abdominal respiration is useful in cases where it can be carried out. Prill also feels that in nature and in man rhythms are of great importance. The respiratory rhythm, he believes, exerts a great influence on the physical and mental condition. Rhythmic activity, for example that of soldiers on the march, can be of great value. Certain emotional states (moaning, sighing, etc.) may be expressed in a change of the rhythm of respiration. The regulation of the respiratory rhythm can equally influence the emotional state of the woman. The appreciation of time is also a function of the rhythm. If this latter is regular, time can appear half as long. He tries to use the respiratory rhythm in order to obtain a general relaxation. Inspiration, he considers, is accompanied by feelings of agitation, of tension and of lightness, and expiration by sensations of 'falling, of relaxing or heaviness.' Respiration produces an alternation between tension and relaxation. In the correct training of the woman a feeling of general relaxation is linked with expiration. Using the expression which Prill employed to broadly represent these views, one can say that the pain ought to be 'expired'. However, he recognizes that this training is not always possible, and particularly so with women who are very tense. He considers that his technique of producing a general relaxation by means of respiration comes very near to the procedures of Read and Heardman. But it should not be forgotten that these two authors have not developed as explicit theoretical considerations as those of Prill.

(b) Autogenous Training

As well as the exercises which have just been described, Schultz's exercises are practised in the sessions and in the home. It is desirable that the pregnant woman should learn the six recommended exercises. The most useful one with regard to childbirth, particularly with regard to hypalgesia, is that respiratory exercise which consists of abandoning oneself to the automatic function of respiration. Contraction is then felt as a sensation of heaviness and of compression in the pit of the stomach. Every woman cannot practise this exercise during childbirth. Certain women can only reach the phases of heaviness and of warmth, during which hypalgesia is still possible. In 66 per cent of his cases Prill adds trilene at the phase of complete dilatation.

(c) Didactic Elements

The didactic part of his practice is based on the book *Childbirth without Fear* and on that of BURGER-EASTMAN, *Die Werdende Mutter* [67]. Instruction is given to small groups consisting of three to five women, as for the exercises. It takes the form of interviews during which the women can discuss their emotional problems. They also establish contact with the doctor and with the other members of the group. Having already seen the importance which Prill attaches to the interpersonal factor, and his emphasis on the autogenous method (indirect action) we shall see, however, that numerous elements appertaining to direct suggestion nevertheless enter into his method in spite of his intention of keeping to the indirect action. Prill criticized the active attitude thought to be so important by the Russians and writes 'the important thing is not to grit the teeth or to be heroic in adopting an active attitude as with the Russians'. He adds that in his method the parturient woman becomes calm and resolute in an attitude of concentrated passivity.

We have described this method at length owing to its being one of the two chief methods of relaxation. Experimentally it is most interesting, but its mass application, like that of hypnosis, would seem difficult. Psychotherapeutic skill on the part of the doctor is essential, and Schultz* insists that the practice of his method must be confined to doctors. Moreover, it introduces added factors which makes the burden of preparation still heavier.

*Personal communication.

CHAPTER 8

HYPNOSUGGESTIVE METHODS IN ANGLO-SAXON COUNTRIES AFTER THE SECOND WORLD WAR

DURING the Second World War, hypnosis proved useful as a rapid psychotherapeutic measure in military psychiatry. Since the war there has been renewed interest in the method in Anglo-Saxon countries, and particularly in the United States. Attempts have been made to use hypnotism in obstetrics.

The first publication was that of KROGER and DE LEE [287] in 1943. It dealt with eleven cases, the first of whom went as far back as 1931, and was chiefly concerned with deep hypnotic states during childbirth, with amnesia. The woman was delivered in a hypnotic state. She was able to talk with the operator, to ask for food, to pass water, and to go to the lavatory as she desired (somnambulism). The relationship could be transferred to the nurse or to the husband who, in the absence of the doctor, were able to direct the woman. In the eleven cases episiotomy was systematically carried out and forceps were used (the current practice in the United States). Some years after this publication by Kroger and de Lee, other papers appeared dealing with hypnosis in obstetrical analgesia: ABRAMSON and HERON [2], NEWBOLD [379–382], KROGER and FREED [285], MICHAEL [366], SCHNECK [495], KROGER [283–285], TRUE [539], KLINE and GUZE [271], DE LEE [119], CLARK [95], AMBROSE and NEWBOLD [13], GREEN [203]. These communications had begun to appear at a time when the interest in psychological analgesia had been reawakened through the spread of Read's method.

The authors simplify the technique of induction. They begin with the premise that hypnosis is a 'continuum', passing from a state of light relaxation to somnambulism. Thus for instance, Abramson and Heron were led to study hypnosis via Read's method. Their reasoning was as follows: Read's method implied education, relaxation and suggestion, and hypnosis also relies on relaxation and suggestion; 'if the Read technique was carried a step further and a trance state induced, the results could be improved' [2].

VOLLMER [569] followed an opposite path. Together with Marsh, he has for several years delivered about sixty women under hypnosis. But they both state that hypnosis is not convenient to practise and that the benefit which resulted was chiefly due to the relaxation. They therefore sought to produce relaxation without hypnosis and thus were led to practise Read's method. From these different papers it is possible to discern the outline of the hypnosuggestive method at present carried out in the United States and Great Britain.

1. PREPARATION

Starting with a state of relaxation an attempt would be made, according to the hypnotizability of the subject, to obtain a trance state of variable depth. It may be that a state of relaxation will be sufficient, relying on suggestibility and the possibility of producing hypnotic phenomena without using 'sleep' ('waking hypnosis', Kroger). In addition, for some writers (MICHAEL [366]) the depth of the trance is not in proportion to the degree of analgesia attained during childbirth. Others are of a different opinion (ABRAMSON and HERON [2], KLINE and GUZE [271]). When deepening the hypnosis, tests of the degree of hypnosis should be avoided (the relationship between the suggested hallucination test and the childbirth could not, for instance, be explained). Newbold uses tests of analgesia to pinprick; other writers (KLINE and GUZE, ABRAMSON and HERON) train the women in autohypnosis.

All the writers give suggestions in the course of preparatory sessions; suggestions of analgesia, of a feeling of lightness of the abdomen, of relaxation (the latter suggestions are also given during contractions), or suggestions directed to substituting the nurse or the husband for the doctor in order to guide the woman during her childbirth. NEWBOLD [379–382] suggests to the woman that during the first phase of labour she will feel the contractions as pleasant sensations, and during the second phase as something to be endured. The sessions begin very early (Newbold). The first two occur at fortnightly intervals, then every month, becoming more frequent before term (at least six sessions in all are given). MICHAEL [366] begins the sessions between the thirty-fourth and the thirty-seventh week of pregnancy. He gives from two to eleven sessions, and states that there is no connection between the number of sessions and the results. Kline and Guze carry out eight individual sessions in all. KROGER [283-285] begins before the seventh month and carries out one session every fortnight. The first session, or the first two, are in general individual and the following are group sessions. Certain writers add didactic elements to the preparation. In Michael's technique the women undergo three courses where they learn the anatomy of the genital organs and physiology of labour.

Educational elements are also found in the work of CLARK [95] of Hollywood. His patients are advised to read the book of Grantly Dick Read *Childbirth without Fear*, or Thoms' book *Understanding Natural Childbirth*. Using a 'Birth Atlas'* he shows them the anatomy and physiology of pregnancy and childbirth. As well as this information he also teaches them the technique of respiration in the different stages, gymnastics and posture training, and gives advice on the postnatal period, breast feeding, care of the breasts, etc. With regard to the hypnosuggestive technique, Clark introduces some innovations. He gives the women, before their preparation, a pamphlet [95, appendix] which aims at conditioning them for hypnosis in the shape of what he calls prehypnotic suggestions. The pamphlet explains how pain, created by tension provoked by fear, can disappear with hypnotic relaxation. The medical uses of hypnosis, and the technique of induction are described.

At the first session, the patient listens to a record made by the doctor, repeating the details in the pamphlet, and adding technical instructions for relaxation. Fifty per cent of the women find themselves in a hypnotic state during this first session. The second session is devoted to training in the technique of relaxation which is described as follows: 'First, muscles are placed under stress. At a given signal, they are released from this stress and simultaneously the attention is detached from the muscles'. During this session 75 per cent of the patients go into hypnosis, without any other form of suggestion. This proportion rises to almost 100 per cent when suggestions of induction of hypnosis are

Birth Atlas, Maternity Center Association, New York, 2nd Ed. 1950.

given at the end of the session. Autosuggestion is also taught, and the women practise this at home several times a day. As well as suggestions with regard to analgesia, the women are given suggestions regarding the postnatal period, concerning lactation, etc.

2. CONDUCT OF CHILDBIRTH

The woman ought to be delivered either in a hypnotic state or in a waking state. She should be hypnotized by the doctor in the labour ward or she should enter a state of autohypnosis pending the arrival of the doctor, sometimes even for the duration of the childbirth. The doctor ought to be able to transfer his suggestive capacity to the interne or nurse so as to space out his own interventions. Certain women are able to follow their deliveries in a mirror (KROGER [283-285]). Suggestions can even be given by telephone* or by gramophone records (Kroger).

Certain writers used drugs only in cases of failure. Others combined their method with the systematic use of medicaments, but in doses which are less than the usual doses necessary to produce analgesia.

3. RESULTS

The use of the method is very limited. The study of Abramson and Heron deals with one hundred cases; Michael with thirty cases and Kline and Guze with twenty-eight. Figures are not given by the other authors. Abramson and Heron who have studied one hundred cases with a control group and who used an analgesic (pethidine), obtained a reduction in medication of 20 per cent; the mean dose was 103·5 mg in the women who had been prepared, instead of 125 mg in the others. With regard to the analgesia, if it is possible to rely on subjective accounts, then it was obtained in all cases. Michael reports that 73 per cent of the women had had a completely painless delivery. He stresses that pregnant women are very hypnotizable and that the volunteers who make up his case material lend themselves very well to the application of the method. Of the thirty women treated by Kline and Guze 57 per cent received no medication, 17 per cent needed less than usual, 23 per cent had a medium dose and three per cent

*A procedure which had already been in use for rehypnotization at the end of the nineteenth century (LIÉGEOIS [331]).

more than the dose. In 67 per cent of cases, either a complete or partial analgesia was obtained by autohypnosis, heterohypnosis or a posthypnotic technique.

CLARK [95] has carried out his method in about 40 per cent of his practice. One-third of the women participating received no medication throughout childbirth and labour (comprising episiotomy, manual exploration of the uterus, examination of the cervix and posterior colporraphy). He had first used Read's method, but later had occasion to use the hypnosuggestive method in several cases where the previous childbirth had been conducted by him following the former method. The majority of these women much preferred hypnosis. 'As they state, the duration of labour seems shorter, there is less fatigue and nervous exhaustion, relaxation is easier and much deeper, an anaesthetic is not required for the episiotomy and the repair, the stitches are not painful, and they have more energy and vitality during the entire recovery period'. All the writers mention the obstetrical and medical advantages reported in all the other psychological methods.

Psychoanalytic concepts have made themselves felt, as is shown by the fact that the personality of the parturient has been taken into consideration. KROGER, for instance, without indicating the number of his cases, has studied the personality of women wanting to undergo either the hypnotic method or the method of Natural Childbirth. He found common traits in both categories, compulsive traits and the desire to please a paternal figure (the obstetrician) [284]. KLINE and GUZE, by means of tests, attempted to evaluate the capacity of the patient to benefit from hypnosis during childbirth. They also avoided patients whose emotional adjustment was too precarious for them to be able to undergo a hypnotic treatment [271].

CHAPTER 9

THE PSYCHOPROPHYLACTIC METHOD IN THE SOVIET UNION*

1. DIRECTION OF THE RUSSIAN MINISTRY OF HEALTH 13 FEBRUARY 1951

BEFORE passing to the history, theory and practice of the method, a detailed summary will be given of the *Temporary Directions on the Practice of the Psychoprophylaxis of the Pains of Childbirth* No. 142, of the Ministry of Health of the Soviet Union, 13 February 1951. This is a basic document, and includes a description of the method; it was published following the Leningrad Conference of January 1951, at which the problem of the psychoprophylaxis of the pain of childbirth had been discussed. It is composed of four parts [38].

(1) The first is an introduction, explaining briefly the general ideas underlying the method, and stressing above all that if the method is to succeed it depends upon the 'instruction, teaching and education of the staff, and the increase in the general and obstetrical knowledge of the staff of the maternity unit'.

In principle each session consists of three parts: (a) medical and obstetrical examinations, (b) theoretical lectures and practical exercises, and (c) 'strengthening' of the analgesiant procedures 'by a constant repetition in a state of "relaxing-rest".'†

(2) Chapter 2 deals with the technique of the preparation. This starts in the thirty-sixth week of pregnancy, and comprises five or six lessons at intervals of three or four days. If necessary the number of sessions can be reduced to three.

---

*After the Kiev Congress of February 1956 the method has been known as 'The Method of Psychoprophylactic Preparation of Pregnant Women for Childbirth'.

†Literally, 'quietness-repose'. It consists of hypnoidal states, states of 'light inhibition', during which suggestibility is increased. 'A reflex-conditioned consolidation of the analgesic effect of the procedures' is thus obtained [559]. This procedure was first applied in all cases but was later reserved only for difficult cases. DONIGUEVITCH [132] gives a detailed description of the procedure. In the French method described by LAMAZE neuromuscular education has replaced this.

The first session is an individual one. It includes a physical examination, an obstetrical examination and a detailed psychological anamnesis, paying regard to any psychic trauma. The conversation is then brought round to woman's fear of childbirth, which the method aims to combat. 'Positive emotions' must be created by exalting the joys of motherhood. The age of the parturient, her education and her profession must all be taken into account.

The second is a group session, as are the remainder. It consists of a part describing the mechanism of childbirth, and another which is psychotherapeutic and educational, aiming at the removal of the belief in the ineluctable nature of the pain in childbirth.

The third and fourth sessions deal with the physiology of the first stage of labour, and with the mother's subjective sensations during this phase. Procedures for reducing the pain are also taught during these sessions. These consist of: (1) deep rhythmical breathing during contractions, (2) abdominal effleurage in a rhythm linked with inspiration and expiration, and (3) pressure on the following points: anterior—anterior superior iliac spine; posterior—surface of the rhomboid muscles. The posterior pressure is applied either by the wrists, or by a hard roller.

The fifth session is devoted to the explanation of the subjective sensations felt by the mother during the second stage of childbirth. She is taught the best posture to take during this phase, and how to co-operate actively in the expulsion.

The sixth session is one of synthesis.

The *Directions* also recommend a rapid preparation for women who have not been prepared based on a good relationship with the staff, a feeling of confidence and a rapid teaching of what her behaviour should be during childbirth. To reassure her, the parturient is put in contact with mothers who had had a successful painless childbirth by the Psychoprophylactic Method.

(3) The third part deals with the organization of the Maternity Unit, and the education of the staff. The medical and nursing staff, as well as the midwives, must be made acquainted, in five lessons, with Pavlov's theories and the Psychoprophylactic Method; for auxiliary staff, three lessons are recommended. A calm and kindly atmosphere is essential in the classroom. In the Maternity Unit, the mothers are followed through from their admission until the end of the birth. Agitated women must be

kept away from the women who have been prepared. Breathing exercises are recommended in the first stage; when dilatation is approaching completion, abdominal effleurage is begun. When dilatation is delayed the third exercise is started. In prolonged labour indirect suggestion is recommended, using injections of glucose-serum or inhalations of oxygen, and telling the mother that they are to relieve pain. When the moment arrives, the mother is told to make the necessary efforts for the expulsion, and she is reminded of the position to adopt for the passage of the head. At the end of the birth the doctor must assess the degree of analgesia based on objective observations of her behaviour (such as her movements, cries, responses) and on statements about her subjective sensations.

(4) The fourth part of the *Directions* describes the method of assessing the results, according to the behaviour of the mother during the first phase of dilatation, the second phase of dilatation and the phase of expulsion, and her statements at the end of the birth.

2. GENESIS OF THE METHOD

Just as hypnosis is found at the origin of all medical psychotherapy, so also is it the source of the Psychoprophylactic Method. The Russian protagonists of the method are unanimous about its origin.

'The new form of verbal analgesia in obstetrics,' writes PLATONOV, 'has come from our hypnosuggestive method' [426]. In the history of psychological obstetrical analgesia VELVOVSKI considers that 'the first stage was the hypnosuggestive method, the second the Psychoprophylactic Method' [558]. At the Leningrad Conference NICOLAIEV declared 'the roots of the Psychoprophylactic Method are found in the principles of our previous hypnosuggestive method based on Pavlov's doctrines' [389]. 'The hypnosuggestive method, the first application of Pavlov's doctrine in obstetrics, is of great theoretical importance; it preceded the new psychoprophylactic tendency' write VELVOVSKI and his collaborators, in the introduction to their book [558].*

*The French publications have either neglected or denied this fact of such importance for the understanding of the method. Lamaze, for instance, wrote 'The Psychoprophylactic Method is quite different from those derived from hypnosis or suggestion' [295]. It is only recently that the role of hypnosis in the genesis of the method has been reconsidered (VERMOREL [561], ECONOMIDES [143]), but ANGELERGUES and ROELENS [17] in 1957 barely mention it.

How has this development come about, this transition from the hypnosuggestive method to the psychoprophylactic method? The answer will give us a better understanding of the fundamental principles of the method. The Russian workers started from an experimental basis, in recognizing the phenomenon of analgesia produced by hypnotic suggestion. This empirical fact proved to them that psychological analgesia was a reality. For 25 years they experimented with the hypnosuggestive method in all its forms, and concluded (PLATONOV [426], VELVOVSKI [558]) that:

(1) Pain is not a necessary accompaniment of childbirth.
(2) Verbal suggestion may have an analgesic effect.
(3) Hypnosis involves no danger to mother or child.
(4) It is possible to use certain variants of suggestion, particularly indirect suggestion.
(5) There are no contra-indications, except in known psychopaths.
(6) The absence of fear and anxiety is a very important factor.

These conclusions formed the basis for the creation of the Psychoprophylactic Method. Velvovski and his collaborators consider that the hypnosuggestive method has provided the foundations of verbal obstetrical analgesia, but 'it has not had a general application in spite of its physiological basis or its great efficacy in individual preparation. This fact has obliged us to seek for new forms of psychotherapy and psychoprophylaxis in obstetrics' [558].

As we have previously seen, elements of psychoprophylaxis were already present in the hypnosuggestive method: teaching, suppression of fear, creation of positive emotions, good relationship between the therapist and the patient, environment of the maternity hospital (Platonov, Chlifer, Kopil-Levina, Zdravomyslov etc. . . .).

It will be seen later that 'hypnosuggestive procedures are also applicable in the psychoprophylaxis of the pains of childbirth' (PLATONOV [427]). The new method (the Psychoprophylactic Method) has the great merit, SALGANNIK believes, of being a technique 'accessible to every doctor and in some extent to the midwife' [485]. The Psychoprophylactic Method arose out of the difficulties in a general application of hypnosis. In the new method the direct suggestion utilized in the hypnosuggestive method disappears in favour of indirect psychotherapeutic means. It was created in 1949 by Velvovski in collaboration with Platonov, Plotitcher and Chougom; Platonov and his pupil, Velvovski, are neuropsychiatrists, Plotitcher and Chougom, obstetricians. It is difficult to understand the fundamentals of the method if its origins and its history are not examined.

In the introduction to their *Psychoprophylaxis of the Pains of Childbirth* [558], we learn from these four authors that 'the Psychoprophylactic Method was created neither in an obstetrical institution nor in a research institute but in a neuropsychiatric department, that of the Ministry of Transport at Kharkov'. For 20 years the doctors of that hospital had particularly concerned themselves with the connections between psychiatry and other branches of medicine. There were small surgical, general medical, and ear, nose and throat departments in this hospital. The project of starting a maternity department there was considered fantastic by some people, but was nevertheless carried through. The collaboration, so difficult to achieve, between psychiatry and other medical specialties bore fruit.

From 1947 on, Velvovski's team began to develop the foundations of a new method, at that time entitled 'Psychotherapeutic Method of Analgesia in Childbirth'. In December 1949 this method had been discussed at Kharkov in a conference consisting of representatives of the Health Services of the Russian Ministries of Transport and Health. Following Nicolaiev's proposal, the method was named 'System of Psychoprophylaxis of the Pains of Childbirth'. From 1950 on, Velvovski, Platonov, Plotitcher and Chougom, began to publish their work. A conference took place at Leningrad from 29 to 31 January 1951 on obstetrical analgesia [99]. This conference was organized by the Academy of Medicine and the Ministry of Health of the Soviet Union, and gathered together obstetricians, neuropsychiatrists and a small number of physiologists (two out of the thirty-nine participants). The first part of the conference was devoted to psychoprophylactic analgesia. The communications of PLATONOV [426], VELVOVSKI [553], and NICOLAIEV [388] dealt with the theoretical problems, others (ASTAKHOV and BESKROVNAIA [23], CHICHKOVA *et al.* [90], KORABELNIK and DARON [280]) presented the practical applications of the method. RAZDOLSKI [455] and GARMACHEVA [186] dealt with the physiological problems of pain. A wide-ranging discussion followed, and disagreement was expressed particularly regarding the theoretical aspects of the methods, much less as to their practical efficacy. Velvovski's method was accepted. Official recognition appeared in the *Directions of the Ministry of Public Health, U.S.S.R.* (No. 142, 13 February 1951) which recommended the Psychoprophylactice Mthod, and which were published a short time after the conference.

Five years after the Leningrad Congress, another congress was held at Kiev from 10 to 14 February 1956, in order to assess the position with regard to the practical application of the method. This congress, to which we will return, led to a change in the name of the method, which was now called 'The Psychoprophylactic Method of Preparation of Expectant Mothers for Childbirth' [100].

3. THEORETICAL ASPECTS

The Psychoprophylactic Method, the result of an empirica evolution of the hypnosuggestive method, was put to practical use without its theoretical basis being really established. The resolution of the Leningrad Congress which officially confirmed the Psychoprophylactic Method, expressly maintained that 'the physiology of the act of childbirth is not sufficiently explored. The Conference considers that there is a grossly insufficient participation of physiologists in the solution of this important problem' [99].

NICOLAIEV, in his closing speech at the same conference, considered that 'the practice, in obstetrical analgesia, is far beyond the theory' and that 'the Psychoprophylactic Method, which has proved itself in practice, has not attained a clear and concise theoretical foundation' and he complains that the obstetricians have not been sufficiently helped by Pavlovian physiologists and neurologists. VELVOVSKI sets up working hypotheses; according to him the method 'is still in the period of elaboration of its theoretical basis' [558]. The resolution of the Kiev Congress declares that 'theoretical researches on the problem of the psychoprophylactic preparation do not account for the practical results. For instance, the mode of action of the psychoprophylactic preparation, the question of the objective evaluation of the analgesic effect, and the importance of the suggestive element have not been sufficiently explained' [467]. All the Russian authors take Pavlovian theory, and the works of Pavlov, Bykov, Ivanov-Smolenski, and others as a basis. Nevertheless, when it comes to the physiological interpretation of the pain of childbirth, and to the mechanism of psychological analgesia, these authors hold different views. Platonov, Velvovski, Nicolaiev and Salgannik are the most important amongst the theoreticians of the Psychoprophylactic Method, and differences exist between them. Salgannik's ideas are often opposed to those of Velvovski; Nicolaiev takes an intermediate position. Amongst others taking part in the theoretical discussions (especially at the Kiev and Leningrad Congresses) were the following workers: BELOCHAPKO [36, 37], DAVIDENKOV [112], ZDRAVOMYSLOV [584], KONSTANTINOV [277], JORDANIA [255], PETROV-MASLAKOV [413].

(a) *Principles Accepted by All Workers*

Some of the fundamental principles of Pavlovian physiology must first be recapitulated. The theory of the conditioned reflex is based on the idea of the temporary connection. The relations of the organism with the external world are mediated by two sorts of reflexes, the absolute or unconditional reflexes, which constitute 'a permanent nervous connection between a given excitant and a well-defined action of the organism' (Pavlov); and the conditional reflexes which constitute 'a temporary nervous connection between one of the numerous events in the outside world and a well-defined activity of the organism' (Pavlov).

The first group of reflexes are controlled by subcortical centres, are inborn, permanent, and form the inheritance of the species. The conditioned reflexes, sited in the cortex, are acquired, temporary and characteristic of the individual. The stimuli from the outer world are continually perceived by the cortex. Each stimulus creates a focus of excitation which is dissipated if it does not connect with other excitatory foci. On the other hand, if a focus already exists, the new focus connects with it and after sufficient repetition can come to participate in the activity of the first one. For instance, if there is a cortical focus of excitement during salivation, caused by presenting meat to a dog, and if this is accompanied several times by the ringing of a bell, the sound stimulus alone can come to produce salivation. This is the simplest example of the conditioned reflex. The signals arriving at the cortex are either of an external, or an internal (visceral) origin. In man there is another group of signals represented by language, and this constitutes the second signalling system.

Reflex-conditioned activity is directed by the interplay of two fundamental processes—excitation and inhibition. These are two antagonist phenomena, constantly interacting, which determine the continuity of the numerous conditioned connections which are being formed. The principal points on which the Russian workers agree are: (1) the dominant role of the cortex in childbirth, (2) its importance in the perception of pain, and (3) the importance of verbal analgesia.

(i) The Role of the Cortex in Childbirth

Pavlov's followers (BYKOV [71], AIRAPETIANTZ [6], KEKTCHEEV and SYROVATKO [263]) have been able to produce conditioned reflexes from the internal organs, and have by so doing established that these organs have a connection with the cortex via receptors. The excitations in these organs are therefore reflected in the cortex; thus the cortex has a functional relationship with the uterus, and uterine function can be influenced by cortical excitation.

(ii) The Role of the Cortex in the Perception of Pain

For the Pavlovian School, pain is undoubtedly the result of cortical function, excitation being transformed into sensation in the cortex by means of a specialized apparatus called an 'analyser'. It is composed of a local receptive organ, transmitting pathways, and a receptor situated in the cortex.

The cortical nature of pain perception is proved by the possibility of forming conditional pain reflexes. The famous experiment of EROFEEVA [150] is cited by all the Russian workers. An electric current is applied to the dog's paw, and provokes a strong withdrawal reaction. The animal also refuses the food given to him. After several repetitions, the animal begins to eat, and finally has no more withdrawal movements after the electric stimulus, but licks his lips; the painful stimulation has been transformed into a 'conditional food excitant'. It is said that Sherrington, watching this experiment, exclaimed 'I can now understand the psychology of martyrs'.

PCHONIK [409, 410] has experimented on man, and was able to transform a subliminal excitation into a painful sensation under the influence of an indifferent stimulus, and vice versa, a painful sensation could be transformed into a subliminal excitation, after association with an indifferent stimulus. It has also been established that speech as well as physical and chemical agents can be used as a stimulus.

Amongst these experiments are the following: the application to the skin of a tube containing water at 63° C induces a painful sensation and a vasoconstriction. If a bell is associated with the painful stimulation, the bell itself and later the sentence 'I ring' will be sufficient to induce the same effect: pain and vasoconstriction. The sentence 'I am applying "hot"' will replace the painful stimulation, through conditioning. A thermal stimulation with water at 43° induces a feeling of warmth, and a vasodilatation. The verbal stimulus 'apply "warm"' will replace the unconditional stimulation. The experiment can be carried further: the painful stimulation (63°), accompanied by the verbal stimulus 'apply "warm"' (usually associated with the 43° stimulation) will not induce a vasoconstriction, but a vasodilatation and a subjective feeling of warmth.

At the recent Kiev Congress, ANOKHINE [19] pointed to the importance of the latest physiological work on the brain stem reticular formation for the understanding of the central formation of the painful sensation. Using modern electrophysiological techniques, MORUZZI and MAGOUN [374] discovered the ascending activating reticular system. Stereotaxic techniques have made it possible to place electrodes in the brain extremely precisely, and by stimulating the region of the reticular formation, Magoun and Moruzzi were able to obtain E.E.G. tracings similar to those found during the transition from sleep to waking ('arousal').

The reticular formation, situated between the medulla and the thalamus, controls the activity of the whole cortex. It controls the waking-sleep cycle, and thus has an important effect on consciousness. The connections between the reticular formation and the cortex are diffuse. Stimulation of the reticular formation at any point activates the whole of the cortex; it is thus a non-specific cortical projection system.*

The reticular formation is linked by collateral pathways to the great sensory tracts, and it is possible that sensory stimuli travel toward the reticular formations through these collateral channels. The stimuli then lose their specificity and activate the reticular formation which, in turn, activates the cortex, putting it into a state of readiness, when it can analyse the sensory messages.

Taking these new data into account, Anokhine drew up a scheme 'for the formation of painful sensation as a subjective state in the central nervous system'. He cites the works of MURPHY and GELLHORN [376] who showed that the painful afferent impulses, before reaching the thalamus, pass through some collateral channels to the reticular formation. He then proceeds as follows: 'A very strong painful impulse reaching the central nervous system provokes an excitation at two levels. First, an excitation of the cerebral cortex occurs corresponding to the local sensation of a stimulus. Then, some 1 m sec later, the same impulse passes through the reticular formation and the hypothalamus, and acts simultaneously on all the parts of the cortex, taking the form of a general and powerful current of excitation. A strong emotional tension then occurs which mobilizes all the reflex-conditioned resources of the cortex. This state of the cortex is considered as the material basis of consciousness, as far as this would appear to be the result of a widespread synthesis of the various aspects of cortical and subcortical activity'. NICOLAIEV [392] considers that Anokhine's ideas are correct and confirms Pavlov's conceptions on the influence of subcortical centres on the cortex.

It would seem that these recent data open up new ground for understanding the difficult problem of the central formation of pain sensation. Analgesia produced by psychological means has been considered so far by the Pavlovian School as resulting from a purely cortical excitation followed by an inhibition, produced by negative induction. Now it may have to be considered in relation to the reticular formation.

*A report on the present state of our knowledge on this whole question has been made recently by BONVALLET [53] and by HUGELIN [238], whose work also provides an important bibliography.

(iii) The Role of Speech

The effect of words on the expectant mother is the basis of the psychoprophylactic method. The Pavlovian School provides a physiological interpretation for the mechanism of this action; speech is a material stimulus just as any other physical stimulus. 'Speech', Pavlov wrote, 'is a real conditioning stimulus, just the same as other stimuli common to men and animals; but it also is quite unique. No qualitative nor quantitative comparison can be made between them. Speech, on account of the life experiences of the adult man, is linked with all the internal or external excitation impinging the cortex—it is their signal, and it replaces them. That is why it can cause the same actions and reactions as these excitations'. Bykov, one of the proponents of cortico-visceral pathology in Russia has also written 'speech can produce extraordinary effects' in the human organism.

Following the French clinicians of the great period of hypnosis, experimental studies were carried out in various countries on the action of verbal suggestion on various functions of the organism. In Russia, Platonov, a pupil of Bechterew, studied the biochemical and trophic modifications that can be produced by verbal suggestion. Given this power of speech, it is possible to understand how analgesia can be produced by verbal action.

(b) The Controversial Problems
(i) The Nature of the Pain of Childbirth

The essential starting point of Velvovski's doctrine, whence arises all his theoretical considerations, is the fact that he believes pain in childbirth is not a physiological phenomenon. Pain is not inherent in the act of childbirth, any more than it exists, for instance, in the act of swallowing or defaecating. Signalization to the cortex of the beginning of the childbirth arises as an interoceptive reflex at a subthreshold level (Bykov). When the process is normal the cortex 'is aware' but does not start its 'emergency mechanisms'. Pain is not felt. Originally VELVOVSKI [553] considered that all the pain of childbirth would be reflex-conditioned. Later on, his attitude became less definite. In 1954 he wrote: 'We have now abandoned our first too elementary conceptions of the reflex-conditioned mechanisms of the origin of the pain of childbirth' and he formulates his present views as follows [558].

The pain of childbirth can arise from two sources: (1) pains with a somatic origin, indicating a pathological state in the uterine region; impulses can arise therefrom which 'bombard' the cortex, pass the subthreshold level, and become painful sensations, thus indicating the physiological difficulties of the birth. And (2) 'psychogenic' or better 'cerebrogenic' or 'functional' pains, which are cortical pains occurring in a physiological childbirth, and arising from a disturbance of the intracortical (between the processes of excitation and inhibition) and cortical-subcortical 'dynamic relations'.

Amongst the intracortical disturbances 'phasic states' (the 'paradoxical state' during which a weak stimulus provokes a strong reaction and vice versa) which increase the already existing cortical inhibition present in every childbirth, play an important part. These 'phasic states' allow the passage of impulses which otherwise would remain at a 'subliminal' level. The cortico-subcortical dynamic state is determined not only by biological factors, but also by psychological ones—fear, 'negative emotions' and beliefs, for example. VELVOSKI [558], who has devoted himself to the study of cortical phenomena, recognizes that he originally underestimated the local factor in pain, but he still believes that intracortical and cortical-subcortical relationships are by far the most important in the perception of pain. The material substrate exists locally, but the higher nervous activity is a factor as 'material' as any other.

Pain sensitivity and pain are not synonymous. The morphological conductors of sensitivity are 'instruments' but not 'musicians' says Velvovski. It is the cortex which 'orchestrates' everything. Excitation can remain at an subliminal level. Velvovski bases his fundamental hypothesis on the nature of the pain of childbirth on the fact that 7–14 per cent of women give birth without pain, even without any preparation. In some peoples, all the women give birth in this way. For instance, in Russia this occurs in certain tribes of Daghestan as well as in some in the Polar regions. He does not deny the existence of pain in animals, but is opposed to the idea of its utility as a 'signal' warning the female to prepare herself for a primordial biological function. This hypothesis was put forward by ELIGULACHVILI [145] in his study of the pain of parturition in monkeys. Velvovski postulates the existence of other 'signals' which are 'obscure sensations', 'badly defined' (using Setchenov's phrase) signals which can make the animal feel the approach of the birth.

He explains the origin of the pain of childbirth in the following manner. At first there were pains of the first group, arising from pathological childbirth in individuals; out of these arose the pains of the second group, caused by neurodynamic modification in the Higher Nervous Activity; there then occurs a generalization of the pain. Velvovski believes that in these remote times the great number of difficult and complicated childbirths was due to early marriage and to the absence of hygiene. The explanation given by the family was of a magical nature; later, religion interpreted it as a punishment for original sin. Man also used this state of affairs to affirm his superiority, in order the better to exploit his wife. Descriptions of painful childbirth in literature have also served to strengthen this idea in the human mind.

Nicolaiev adopts a less definite attitude with regard to the nature of the pain of childbirth. He does not consider that pain is always 'pathological', but he does not believe that pain is inevitable. There is a material physiological basis for the pain; there are mechanical changes in the genital organs, and vascular and humoral modifications in the woman which act on the pain receptors; these modifications can be felt as sensations of heaviness, or of tension, and not necessarily as pain. Sensations become painful when factors of an emotional or reflex-conditioned order are added. Pains are therefore determined by anatomico-functional causes (but not necessarily pathological), or by neurodynamic disturbances or by both together. Nicolaiev criticizes Velvovski for having laid too much stress on the cortex, and for underestimating the action of the subcortical region on the cortex. He believes, with Pavlov, that the action of the subcortical centres on the cortex is more important than the opposite one. But he agrees that Velvovski and his co-authors were correct in drawing attention to the importance of cerebral neurodynamic relationships, but considers as dualistic the dichotomy into 'somatic' and 'psychogenic' pain.

For SALGANNIK [483, 484] the pain of childbirth is a physiological phenomenon. Receptors and analysers of pain exist which do not come into action—as Velvovski believes—only in pathological childbirth, or under the influence of fear. Pain is unthinkable without the cortex, but it cannot exist without an impulse coming from the particular receptor. Pain, as a subjective sensation, appears at the same time as the contraction and disappears with it. He quotes the case of two women having lesions of the spinal cord, who although they were frightened, felt nothing of their childbirth. He criticizes Velvovski for invoking the idea, borrowed from Bykov, of the interoceptive subliminal reflex. He believes that it has no relation to pain, which can only arise with the participation of the cortex. The pain of childbirth is a 'mixed pain, both somatic and visceral, the visceral part prevails in the first phase of the birth, and the somatic one in the second phase'. Furthermore, impulses also come from the baroreceptors, chemoreceptors and receptors from the uterine vascular system, all of which give a particular 'coloration' to the pain of childbirth [484]. On this anatomico-functional foundation, Salgannik admits the existence of emotional stratifications showing 'complex groups of conditional and unconditional reflexes'. This emotional factor 'complicates the pain of childbirth, and gives it its particular form' [484]. Salgannik points out that animals suffer, and he believes that pain has played an active part in phylogenesis by obliging the animal to find a safe place in which to give birth.

BELOCHAPKO [36] does not admit a parallel between the act of childbirth and other physiological functions. Childbirth only occurs a few times in life, and mechanical distension is never as great as during childbirth. DAVIDENKOV [112] criticizes the misuse of the term 'reflex-conditioned pain', and doubts whether such a pain can exist in childbirth. He gives an example—if a prick is associated with a light, the light alone will later be able to produce pain. This pain is reflex-conditioned pain. But he adds 'I very much doubt if this mechanism can take place in childbirth. If the pain is associated with the total surroundings, why does the pain disappear after the birth?' Nor does he believe in the 'reflex-conditioned, pain-reducing complexes elaborated in the preparation', and he writes 'This constitutes a training of cortical function in a certain direction; but where is the method of conditioned reflexes? It seems to me that it does not exist'.

At the Kiev Congress (1956) an even greater reaction took place against the supremacy of reflex-conditioned events in the genesis of the pain of childbirth. For instance KONSTANTINOV [277] strongly criticized the dualistic position of Velvovski, who distinguishes a pain of cortical origin in a physiological birth, and a pathological pain of peripheral origin. He does not consider that childbirth is a physiological event, like other physiological happenings, for they do not involve a risk of cervical tears, massive haemorrhages and other complications. He considers that the 'primary sources of the pain of childbirth are peripheral painful stimulations, without making any distinction between a physiological or pathological childbirth. Therefore the pain-reducing effect of the psychoprophylactic preparation must be considered as due to an anaesthesia of the local receptors, artificially created. This does not deny the importance of functional relations in the central nervous system'.

JORDANIA [255] considered that there are two types of pain; unconditional (somatic) and reflex-conditional. PETROV-MASLAKOV [413] spoke of two components of the pain, one 'unconditional, arising especially at the beginning of the childbirth, of a visceral type of pain; the other, reflex-conditioned. . . .'

(ii) State of the Cortex during Childbirth

One of the premises of Velvovski's system is the fact that the cortex is in a state of inhibition during the childbirth. He relies on the following facts: the behaviour of the woman very often resembles neurotic behaviour of a 'hysteroidal' type; she sometimes falls into a twilight state—sometimes the reflexes are increased (Babinski, Oppenheimer and Rossolimo). Childbirth does not begin in deep sleep, but on awakening or in the phase of going to sleep; the majority of births occur during the night. He believes, with Ivanov-Smolenski, that the 'cerebral cortex is in a state of inhibition during the realization of an unconditional reflex' [558].

Salgannik finds Velvovski's statements contradictory, when he maintains that the cortex is in a state of inhibition during childbirth, and at the same time directs the process of birth. Davidenkov believes that it is an abuse of Pavlovian terminology to mention phasic states of the mother's cortex. In the paradoxical phase, weak stimuli produce strong reactions, and vice versa. This phase is spoken of when weak stimuli coming from the uterus cause strong perceptions. It ought, therefore, to be possible 'to suppress the pain by strong stimuli coming from the uterus, and this is not the case'.

(iii) Principle of the Method—Cortical Activation

Accepting the fact that, according to Velvovski, pain in a normal childbirth is not a physiological phenomenon, the problem then is not to relieve the pain, but to prevent it. Hence the name of the method 'Psychoprophylaxis of the Pains of Childbirth', or more briefly 'The Psychoprophylactic Method'. The cortex already being in a state of inhibition during the childbirth, the Psychoprophylactic Method does not produce an inhibition (which occurs during hypnosis and suggestion), but a 'cortical activation', which is obtained by means of education, instruction, teaching and the use of pain-reducing procedures. It is concerned with the suppression of the 'phasic state' in which the cortex finds itself during childbirth.

Velvovski believes that in the hypnosuggestive method, an analgesia but not a prophylaxis is obtained. The Psychoprophylactic Method must aim at 'annihilating' the pain of childbirth as a socio-biological factor. He believes that the hypnosuggestive methods are therapeutic methods, and, as the pain of childbirth is not an illness, therapy is unnecessary. With hypnosis, which produces an inhibition, the pain is treated, but in fact, it must be prevented. Psychotherapy of a more major type only begins when a pathological condition is uncovered during the Psychoprophylactic Preparation. According to Velvovski, activation is based on what he calls 'the second therapeutic principle', which is excitation. The first principle is protective inhibition, the basis of sleep treatment or hypnotherapy. 'If inhibition possesses a powerful therapeutic action, excitation must be, in certain circumstances, just as efficient', he writes. Petrova proved this pharmacologically, by using a bromide-caffeine mixture. When the cortex is activated, impulses remain on the subliminal level and cannot be transformed into painful sensations. The same result is obtained by the 'analgesic procedures, which are meant to stimulate the state of wakefulness of the cortex, and to bring it to an active state, to "corticalization".'

Velvovski's hypotheses would seem to lack clarity and are

difficult to prove. According to him there are two mechanisms leading to the suppression of pain, in the first an analgesia results from inhibition, in the second prophylaxis would occur as a result of an elevation of the cortical threshold to pain. Nicolaiev believes that two states cannot be opposed in the cortex, one 'active' and one 'inhibited', these states, resulting from a process of excitation and inhibition only represent parts of a whole. He cites Pavlov, who writes that 'the process of excitation is closely linked with that of inhibition; when excitation weakens, inhibition in its turn also disappears'.

Some reservations must be made when speaking of 'activation'. This activation is very relative; it is better to 'speak of the necessity of forming new positive conditioned reflexes. One must speak of transforming the reflexes, and of stopping unnecessary ones, which hinder the correct development of the birth'. Nicolaiev continues: 'Platonov and the other authors of the psychoprophylactic method consider that it is indispensable for the prophylaxis of pain to free the cortex from inhibition and its paradoxical states, by means of cortical activation. However, the promoters of the psychoprophylactic method confuse the different factors in their own method, and the times at which they occur, and this leads to a confusion of ideas. A very definite differentiation must be made: Preparation of expectant mothers by the Psychoprophylactic Method is one thing and the attitude of the woman during the childbirth is another. The conditions of the teaching given to the expectant mothers for preparing them for their painless childbirth doubtless contributes to a certain inhibition of the cortex, and to the creation of hypnoidal phases. This state of the cortex is not yet hypnosis, but it is no longer a state of absolute wakefulness, the active state of the cortex. And in this state, the suggestions which represent such an indispensable element for any teaching and any education, and which are temporary connections only, are more strongly fixed by the cortex. A deep hypnosis, or a deep inhibition, spreading widely, is not absolutely necessary for the firm fixation and realization of these suggestions. We also know that the first phases of the state of inhibition are enough to obtain this effect. We can, therefore, suppose that while undergoing a course of training in the Psychoprophylactic Method, the cortex of the patients is really in a state of inhibition. During childbirth, the cortex must be active, but in the sense of a normalization of cortical-subcortical relations, and of an optimum correlation between the fundamental processes of excitation and inhibition' [390].

Salgannik proposes that 'activation' should not be overstressed because if exaggerated, it can produce an imbalance between excitation and inhibition. Phasic states or hypnoidal states are not negative effects only but also positive, as these states are favourable to the extinction of reflexes related to the pain. In certain cases he even advises the use of hypnotic sleep, in order to consolidate the process of preparation. In other cases, when the woman is not accessible to teaching, recourse can be made to hypnoidal states, and even hypnotic sleep can be used. 'Our observations prove,' he writes, 'that the passage to the hypnoidal state and to hypnotic sleep can sometimes be obtained very easily by means of the same "exercises", having the same verbal content, but taking a more direct and insistent action' [485]. The essential feature of the Psychoprophylactic Method is 'the influence by speech, persuasion, and verbal suggestion'. The field of action of language is extremely large, varying from speech divested of meaning, to hypnosis.

Zdravomyslov considers that in the hypnosuggestive method, as he practises it, there is no inhibition during childbirth, as the great majority of the mothers give birth in a waking state (887 out of 1000) [584]. At the Kiev Congress DOLINE and SALGANNIK [131] also severely criticized Velvovski, maintaining that in psychoprophylaxis 'one of the most important physiological mechanisms is the process of active inhibition, capable of abolishing the painful reactions occurring during the childbirth' (the pain of childbirth is considered as a physiological phenomenon by these authors).

NICOLAIEV [394] tried again, in 1957, to formulate the problem taking into account these criticisms. His report is not very clear; we retain only what follows: The Psychoprophylactic Method has an action on the two major processes of cerebral activity, excitation and inhibition. The analgesic effects are produced by several mechanisms. The preparation creates foci of excitation which either block the stimuli, or suppress those which surmount the threshold. This suppression occurs either by active conditioned inhibition, or by inhibition following negative induction.

(iv) The Role of Suggestion

Velvovski admits that there is a little suggestion in all the essentials of the Psychoprophylactic Method, but he assigns it less importance than do Nicolaiev, Salgannik and others. Platonov believes that there are many elements of suggestion in the teaching, but these elements are on a different level 'superior in quality'. His pupil Velvovski thinks that the difference is essential—suggestion cannot be compared in the two cases. He believes that in therapeutic suggestion, the subject is passive and suggestibility increases with the degree of inhibition. In the teaching however, there is no passivity on the part of the pupil, the teacher's success is greater 'when the pupil is active and critical' [558]. The aim of the pain reducing procedures is to maintain the cortex on guard, to 'corticalize' the mother. It is difficult to understand the difference between the physiological mechanisms when the 'procedures' are used as indirect suggestion, or when they are used in the psychoprophylactic method.

Moreover, in 1951, Velvovski did not differentiate between the physiological mechanisms of 'corticalization' by the 'procedures', and of indirect suggestion. He wrote 'Indirect suggestion in this case is a real motor activity which creates a focus of excitation in the cortex, brings the cortex to an active state, protects it from an excessive negative induction, and creates conditions by which impulses arising from the birth, and coming from lower levels, will remain below the cortical threshold, and will remain there so as not to be transformed into pain' [553].

His attitude is different in his later formulation. Discussing the views of Davidenkov, who believes that activation 'settles the pain according to the principle of negative induction', Velvovski considers that the procedures employed in the previous methods had as their aim an indirect suggestion (combined excitation and inhibition) but that their use in the psychoprophylactic method 'follows another aim, using a different principle', which consists essentially in a slight excitation of the cortex (prophylaxis by an elevation of the threshold). Indirect suggestion lessens the pain, but the procedures of the Psychoprophylactic Method do not have to do this, as the pain must not be allowed to appear [558]. In his survey on the practical application of the Psychoprophylactic Method, PLOTITCHER [430] admits that the 'procedures' have two modes of action, depending on the particular case: (1) activation of the woman's cortex can avoid the beginning of the pain by maintaining the stimulation at a subthreshold level (prophylactic action), and (2) if pain appears, the procedures create a focus of cortical excitation, which according to the law of induction, exerts an inhibitory action on the other regions of the cortex (therapeutic action).

Plotitcher gives his explanation in terms of reflexology and cites for his purpose the following passage from Pavlov: 'A reflex takes place; this means that there is an excitation in a given point of the central nervous system. If, at the same time, another reflex takes place, this means that another excitation takes place at another part of the central nervous system, then the first reflex weakens or else disappears completely. It can be imagined that during the production of the second reflex, energy is drawn away from the first centre, and directed on the new centre, and its manifestation weakens or disappears completely if this diversion is very substantial'.

In order to obtain activation of the cortex, or a focus of excitation, the character of the exercises does not matter; for example, attention is mobilized by timing the intervals between the contractions; or respiration is used, or other movements.

Concerning suggestion, Nicolaiev writing in the conclusions of the reports on the Leningrad Conference, says, 'Elements of suggestion are found in the new Psychoprophylactic Method, and this is normal, because it concerns a verbal action on man. This must not be denied, nor should one be afraid of it!' He believes that Velvovski minimizes the importance of suggestion. 'Can teaching and instruction be opposed to suggestion and vice versa?' He believes, with Pavlov, that 'suggestion is the simplest and the most typical of the conditioned reflexes of man' and even that 'these notions of education, instruction, teaching, suggestion, are identical from the physiological point of view' [390].

Salgannik admits that suggestion plays a large part in the Psychoprophylactic Method. Suggestion exists at all stages of the preparation, whether in the educational component, or in the 'procedures'. He thinks that the mode of action of suggestion, or influence by speech is very widespread. An action on the cortex, of varying degree, from the creation of limited foci of excitation, with extinction of certain reflexes, and limited inhibition, up to deep sleep with large areas of inhibition, can be obtained by suggestion or by the influence of speech. The manner of speaking, the stereotyped repetition, the atmosphere during the session, all this is very important.

Whilst not denying the importance of the didactic element in the preparation, KONSTANTINOV [277] believes that 'the essential in psychoprophylaxis is suggestion (direct or indirect)'. The woman comes, not to learn, but to suppress her pains. Understanding does not bring analgesia, it is the teaching which 'gives such great possibilities for verbal action on the woman'.

(v) Role of the Nervous Types

The chief problem of the Psychoprophylactic Method is to obtain criteria for predicting a painful childbirth, and for the success of verbal action. Russian workers have attempted, following Pavlov, to classify people according to their 'Nervous Type' (they partially return to the Hippocratic classification). These Nervous Types have been identified by Pavlov in animals (according to the strength and mobility of the process of excitation and inhibition and their balance). Four types have been recognized. The strong, balanced slow type (phlegmatic), the strong, balanced quick type (sanguine), the strong, unbalanced type (choleric), and the weak type (melancholic).

However, in man the problem is complicated by the second signalling system (language) and intermediary types may exist in which the first or second system is predominant (the artistic type, or the intellectual type). Many transitory categories exist. Furthermore, in man, the social is stronger than the biological; the Nervous Type can be transformed as a result of the reactions of the individual to his surroundings. Pavlov considers that the formation of the Type of Nervous System depends on 'education or learning in its widest meaning'. The study of the Nervous Type cannot therefore be considered alone but must be integrated into a historical study of the individual.

Velvovski believes that in a normal childbirth, the Nervous Type of the woman does not matter; it only matters when childbirth is pathological. He stresses the complexity of this problem for many dimensions are to be taken into account: strength—weakness; mobility—inertia; equilibrium between the processes of excitation and inhibition, equilibrium between the first and the second signalling systems. While recognizing the importance of the Nervous Types, he cannot recommend their particular study in practical obstetrics today as they have not yet been standardized. Experience has shown him that the study of the Nervous Type does not enable one to prejudge the results obtained with the method—DAVIDENKOV is also of the same opinion [558].

Nicolaiev considers that Velvovski has under-estimated the problem, and lays more stress on the appreciation of the Nervous Type of the woman, but considers however that the method is as yet incomplete. It will be seen in the chapters dealing with the application of the method, how Nicolaiev and his pupils put their ideas into practice. On the other hand, Salgannik is closer to Velvovski, as, according to him, this question is still poorly understood in man. Women of a 'weak' Nervous Type are seen behaving in the same way as women of a 'strong' Nervous Type and vice versa. Moreover, behaviour is not always in line with the subjective sensation. For instance, stable women with well-developed excitatory processes have strong subjective feelings, but as they also have well-developed inhibition processes, they remain calm.

4. PRACTICAL APPLICATION

The Psychoprophylactic Method is still in a state 'of experimentation, verification, and above all, of improvement' (SALGANNIK [485]. 'Its technique is of a provisional nature' (PLOTITCHER [430]). Since the publication of *Direction No.* 142 in 1951, numerous works have appeared dealing with the problem of Psychoprophylaxis. Six books have been devoted, in large part, to this problem. Three appeared in 1953—one by PETROV-MASLAKOV and ZATCHEPITZKI [415]; one by NICOLAIEV [392]; and a third by SALGANNIK [485]; in 1954, the book by BELOCHAPKO and FOI [38], as well as a collective work by the authors of the method: VELVOVSKI *et al.* [588]. The book by DONIGUEVITCH [132] was published in 1955, and in 1957 a pamphlet by KIRITCHENKO [266] appeared. Many papers have also appeared.

Direction No. 142 is the basic document on the method—

details have been added later in a *Methodological Letter* from the Ministry of Public Health, dated 4 August 1954, which was addressed to all obstetricians. Finally, some modifications were also formulated at the recent Kiev Congress [100]. But the essential structure of the method remains unchanged. Two parts can be distinguished: preparation for childbirth and the childbirth itself.

(a) Preparation

Plotitcher, the co-author of the Psychoprophylactic Method describes five principal factors [430].

(1) Careful somatic examination.

(2) A persuasive action on the mother (insisting on the physiological nature of childbirth, and on the fact that pains are not inevitable).

(3) Suppression of fear. Plotitcher distinguishes between 'sthenic' emotions, which increase the vital tonus of the organism, and 'asthenic' emotions which have the opposite effect, leading to a disturbance of cortical-subcortical equilibrium, and having repercussions on the correct functioning of all bodily activities. Fear is one of the 'asthenic' emotions.

(4) Pain-reducing procedures.*

(5) Educational action: through frequent repetitions, a sort of 'training' is obtained.

(i) Indications

At the beginning, the Psychoprophylactic Method was used in normal childbirth. Today however no contraindications exist for psychoprophylactic preparation; pathological labours simply require a more detailed preparation, and women with psychiatric complications need an individual preparation. These different modalities will be discussed later (p. 129).

(ii) Personnel Employed in the Method

According to Plotitcher, in leading hospitals the responsibility for organizing the preparation can be assigned to a doctor

---

*No English word gives the exact meaning of the Russian word 'priom'. It is translated here chiefly as 'procedure', but sometimes by 'manipulations' or by 'exercises'.

specially chosen for this task, and he will need a special room. The preparation can also be carried out by the obstetrician in his surgery, and this allows a contact between the mother-to-be and her physician from the start. In smaller institutions, a midwife can help the physician. The first session is given by the physician in the presence of the midwife, and the following ones by the midwife under the supervision of the physician. Where there is no doctor, and the midwife delivers the child, she will also carry out the preparation.*

Since the Kiev Congress, the midwife's role is becoming more important. In Kiev, since 1955, she carries out the whole preparation, under the control of the Head of the Department or Clinic, and the post of Teaching-midwife has been created. LOURIE [334], chief obstetrician at the Health Ministry in the Ukraine, who recommended this, gave the following reasons: 'daily experience has shown that preparation gave good results when the physician worked with enthusiasm and belief, when there were elements of suggestion, when there was a good integration between work in out-patients and the wards'. These conditions are best fulfilled by the midwives, rather than by the physicians, who are either too busy or lack interest in the work of preparation.† At the beginning of Lourie's work, the first session was given by the physician, the following ones by the midwives. Later, however, all the sessions were directed by the midwives, the physician coming only at the end in order to control it.

The experience at Kiev was very successful, 70–80 per cent of the mothers could be dealt with, and given four sessions of the Psychoprophylactic Method. In maternity clinics of more than 60 beds, posts of Anaesthetist-midwives were created, and these women were given responsibility for all questions of anaesthesia. In research Institutions, however, preparation must be carried out only by physicians.

NICOLAIEV [393] wonders who ought to carry out preparation: all obstetricians, or specially trained physicians? He believes that the preparation is better carried out by one person only, chosen

---

*A midwife—N. KIRITCHENKO [266]—published in 1957 a pamphlet for the use of training midwives. It contains the text of four sessions of preparation, couched in simple language.
†Thoms has similar ideas [563].

for the following qualifications: great experience, abilities for teaching and communicating, and interest in the work. Where midwives take part in the preparation, Nicolaiev maintains that the first and last sessions be given by a physician. The midwives always play an auxiliary part. In pathological cases, the preparation must always be carried out by the physician.

(iii) The Sessions

Direction No. 142 advised five or six sessions; PLOTITCHER [430] recommends six. They begin at the thirty-fifth week of the pregnancy; preparation must be finished eight days before the expected date of delivery. The *Methodological Letter* of the Ministry of Health in 1954 recommended that the work of psychoprophylactic preparation should begin with an individual approach from the first prenatal consultation; it reduced the number of sessions to four, at the end of the pregnancy (thirty-fifth to thirty-sixth week). This question was raised at the Kiev Congress [90]; it was considered that the reduction in the number of sessions had been unsuccessful, and that there should be a return to five or six sessions.

The Vice-Minister of Public Health in Russia, CHOUPIK [84], had observed that a reduction of the preparation to two or three sessions had been carelessly made. It had often been motivated in order to impress, or else by a degree of carelessness amongst the staff, which brought a risk of discredit to the method. It was true that Belochapko and Petrov-Maslakov had obtained just as good results with both complete and rapid preparation. But the Vice-Minister did not consider these results sufficient proof. A complete preparation, for statistical purposes, must comprise at least four sessions. Kiritchenko also recommends four sessions in her recent pamphlet for training midwives [266].

Rapid methods can no doubt be efficient if they are directed by specially qualified people, but it is clear that for the method in general, a complete preparation is the most efficient.

We shall now proceed to the detailed description of the sessions, following essentially Plotitcher, co-author of the method.

First session.—This is the most important session as it determines the line to be followed in the ensuing preparation. The interview must be held in an atmosphere of calm and patience.

'The expectant mother must be favourably impressed by the attention and the interest of the physician, his kindness, and the understanding he shows of the thoughts and feelings of the mother, and of all the events of her private life'.

This first session includes: (1) a history, both somatic (general and obstetrical), and psychological, (2) a psychotherapeutic part, aiming at the suppression of fear and apprehension, and (3) an orientation toward the continuation of the preparation (group preparation or individual sessions, possibly also therapeutic, somatic or psychological procedures).

The examination takes first the form of an introductory interview designed to establish contact with the mother, a contact essential for going further into the history of the patient, and for all the future preparations. Here are the contents of the interview, allowing for variations according to the intelligence of the mother. All the questions which she may ask must be answered in an intelligible way.

Introductory Interview: 'You have been sent here to us to prepare for painless childbirth. The preparation creates favourable conditions for a normal confinement. If any complications in the pregnancy should appear in the course of this preparation, it will be remedied before the birth. For a month you will come to the out-patients five or six times. There you will be taught how to behave during your labour, how this takes place, and you will be convinced that there is no reason to be afraid. During the confinement the physician will look after you, in order to obtain a correct and painless birth. To do this, your behaviour is very important. Therefore, this behaviour will be taught to you. During the confinement a great deal is up to the woman herself. According to her behaviour, she can keep up her strength or become exhausted for no reason. She must correctly perform exercises which help the confinement.

'It can be said: childbirth is a job, and this job can either be done properly, in the sense of a rapid and happy accomplishment, or incorrectly, by prolonging it and by increasingly useless efforts. An educated man will do his work quicker and with a smaller amount of energy than an ignorant man.

'For a pregnant woman, to learn is not only to learn how to behave; we shall inform you also of what happens during the confinement, and you yourself will be able to feel it and observe it. These instructions will free you from a fear which has no basis, and which is only linked with the expectation of the unknown; this knowledge will bring you calm and confidence.

'In our next interview, we shall come back to this problem in a more complete way. At the moment let us say this: a normal confinement can and must be painless if it is correctly undertaken.'

Physical anamnesis: When the interview is finished, the history is taken again, not only for the usual information, but with special regard to:

(1) *The age of the mother.* Special tact will be necessary for the obstetrical examination of young expectant mothers who have never been previously examined.

(2) *Diseases.* It is necessary to reassure mothers suffering from diseases developed before the pregnancy (cardiovascular, etc.) with regard to the fears they might have about confinement.

(3) *Menstruation.* A late menarche, or a certain general hypoplasis may be a presage of a prolonged confinement.

(4) *Previous confinements.* Previously complicated confinements (difficult presentations, prolonged labour, uterine inertia, forceps application, etc.) may lead to apprehension concerning the next confinement. Naturally, these apprehensions must not be communicated to the mother. Although in general a new confinement is easier than a previous one, the memory of a painful birth can, by a reflex-conditioned mechanism, make the next one just as painful.

(5) *Genito-urinary disorders.* Inflammations, surgical interventions, etc., which have left scars may result in a cervical dystocia.

Psychological examination (details of the nervous system and Higher Nervous Activity): The emotional attitude of the mother toward pregnancy and childbirth is studied. Negative attitudes must be pointed out, their causes found and then corrected. In cases where these negative attitudes take on a *neurotic* character, the women will need an individual approach.

The study of the Nervous Type is always difficult. In large hospitals elaborate methods may be used but the results obtained are of only relative value. For hospitals or clinics which do not have such means, the physician will content himself with biographical information. He will use it to note the strength and the stability of the nervous processes, and the balance between excitatory and inhibitory processes. He will be guided by the following questions.

(1) Emotional development; the woman is asked to talk about any significant events which occurred in her childhood, at school, during adolescence, at the time of her marriage.
(2) Traumatizing events.
(3) Married life and family; principal role in the family.
(4) Professional activity.
(5) Adaptation to new tasks.
(6) Reaction to life difficulties and the ways of overcoming them.

Psychotherapeutic part. Suppression of the fear: In Plotitchen's experience 83 per cent of women experienced fear in relation to confinement. In 30 per cent the fears were more-or-less realistic; in 70 per cent it resulted from either unhappy life experiences (descriptions of painful childbirths by parents, friends, or in books), or from an undetermined source (for instance the woman says 'I feel an unreasonable fear' or else 'I feel as if I will go into the hospital, but never come out of it').

The fears are as follows: fear of the pains, of an abnormal confinement, of surgical intervention, of being torn, of death, of dangers to the child, of a puerperal infection, etc. The intensity of these fears varies, sometimes it is present intermittently, sometimes permanently.

The emotional state of the woman can be influenced in three ways: (1) information and persuasion; (2) the creation of 'positive emotions' linked with maternity; and (3) teaching of anatomy and physiology, and familiarization with the subjective sensations of the different phases of the confinement. The elements of surprise and the unknown are thus suppressed.

These methods are enough for the majority of women, either when limited to one interview, or more, but there is a type of woman for whom this is not enough, and who needs special psychotherapeutic methods.

Second Session.—The principal theme of the second session is: 'Confinement as a normal physiological act is not necessarily linked with organic lesions, that is why it can and must be painless'. The aim is to remove the idea that organic changes accompany the pains. The women must be taught that there is a continuous biological process of adaptation, which serves to prevent the development of lacerations. The mothers are given an elementary lesson on the anatomy of the female organs, and are told in a very simple way the physiology of pregnancy. It is stressed that seven to fourteen per cent of the women give birth naturally, without pain; moreover, in some cases, women feel so little pain, that they only experience the very last phase of childbirth. The results obtained at the clinic, and statements from women having had a painless childbirth are read out, and it is stressed how important is the behaviour of the woman during the confinement.

Teaching on the Higher Nervous Activity is reserved for women of a higher cultural level (doctors, biologists, teachers). 'Using physiological language, the state of the nervous system at the end of the pregnancy and the beginning of the confinement, a state in which there is subcortical excitation, and a cortical inhibition, will be briefly described to the patients. The inhibited cortex reacts to stimulation differently than the 'alert' cortex. Weak signals, which, in an 'alert' cortex would remain below the threshold of frank sensations, can, in an inhibited cortex, be perceived as very strong and painful'.

This same group of women will be told that emotions, and especially fear and other negative emotions, can change the sensitivity to pain. They will be told that the Psychoprophylactic Method is framed so as to act on the Higher Nervous Activity, which plays the most important part in sensitivity to pain.

For women of average cultural level, the data will be largely schematic. Moreover, every possible explanation is given to demolish any incorrect ideas the women have developed, which may provoke pain. For women of a simple cultural level, the teaching must always be accompanied by pictures and concrete comparisons.

KIRITCHENKO [266] makes no mention of Pavlov in her pamphlet, which contains the text of the four lessons given to the pregnant women.

Third and fourth sessions.—The third and fourth sessions deal with the physiology of the first stage of childbirth and with the explanation of subjective sensations, that is to say, the first contractions. These can be felt as a tightening, a pressure or a tension. The mother will be able to note, with a watch in her hand, the intervals between the contractions, and their duration. They must recognize that when regular contractions appear they must go to the hospital without delay.

Pain reducing procedures are taught. They are of two types: (1) Procedures which are of no obstetrical significance, serving to maintain cortical tonus: rhythmical respiration, abdominal effleurage, massage; and (2) postures which are of use during the confinement: relaxation of the smooth muscles and active collaboration in the expulsive efforts.

The first procedure: rhythmical respiration: Breathing slowly, inspiration through the nostrils, expiration by the mouth. This must be used in the first part of the confinement, as soon as the woman feels unpleasant sensations.

Second procedure: abdominal effleurage: carried out when the cervix is three fingers dilated. During the contraction, the woman strokes the skin of the abdomen with the top of her fingers, from the midline to the iliac fossa during slow inspiration, and in the opposite direction during a quicker inspiration (two or three inspirations during one contraction). The hand describes a sort of circle, starting from the midline, passing externally and downwards, and then upwards to close the circle. The woman is instructed as follows: for a stronger contraction, a wider movement and deeper inspiration.

Third procedure: pressure on pain reducing points: This is applied when the former procedure loses its efficacy. During the abdominal pains, pressure is put on the anterior-superior iliac spine: for lumbar pains, pressure is put on the outlines of the rhomboid muscles. It is applied at the same time as a deep inspiration. The pressure on the posterior points is made with the wrists, or with a hard roller. These procedures must not only be taught and explained, but also practised during the training period. The woman's attention must be concentrated on the carrying out of these exercises, in all their details.

Apart from these three principal procedures, Plotitcher recommends other medical and physiotherapeutic measures based on the same physiological mechanisms: 'Kiparski's pencil' (made with menthol and wax, and producing a sensation of cold when applied to the abdomen), dry cupping, blue light, abdominal friction with a mixture of ether and oil, and spraying of ether on the abdominal skin.

The mother is warned that the 'exercises' will be directed by the doctor or the midwife, but she is allowed to practise the first exercise herself (respiration). The other exercises must begin under the direction of the midwife or doctor. The aim of these 'procedures' is to raise the threshold to pain by a cortical activation. But when pain does appear, they stop it by creating a focus of excitation, accompanied by inhibition.

These mechanisms are explained to the mothers according to their cultural level. For instance the simplest example which Plotitcher mentions is as follows: 'You hurt your head. Immediately you rub the place you hurt. This rubbing, this massage, stops the pain. This massage is used in medicine'.

KIRITCHENKO [266] explains to the women that the procedures are aimed at preventing or lessening or suppressing pain. She tells them that if they concentrate their attention on the procedures they will find that the contractions are quicker and less painful. Respiration 'diminishes disagreeable sensations, helps the work of the heart and insures foetal oxygenation' (Plotitcher does not mention these last two points). The mode of action of abdominal effleurage is explained by the same author, on the basis of the correspondence between cutaneous sensibility and the sensibility of certain internal organs.

Fifth session.—This comprises the preparation up to the second stage of the childbirth. It starts with an elementary lesson on the physiology of the second stage, and the sensations which the woman will feel during it. Her attention will be particularly directed to the moment when the head passes the cervix, the second critical moment when pains may occur (the first one being at the end of the period of dilatation).

During this stage, preparation must consist chiefly in training with regard to her behaviour. The woman is told which is the best posture to adopt in the expulsive phase, and how to push and to breathe; breathing in deeply, without breathing out immediately, closing the glottis. She must push, without breathing out, as during defaecation, for as long as possible. When she cannot hold her breath any longer, she blows out, then takes a breath again, and so on, as long as contractions are coming. Two exercises are recommended for this purpose during the preparation. The mother is shown how to keep her glottis closed, by having to stop in the middle of expiration, with her mouth open. She is also taught to hold her breath for as long as possible; if she cannot hold it for more than 10 or 15 seconds, gymnastic exercises are demonstrated as follows: (1) the woman stands up, arms by the side, feet apart, arms raised above the head, and breathing in. (2) Arms brought back to the side, with breathing out.

She is advised to carry out this exercise at home for ten minutes each day.

The woman must also be taught how to relax her sphincters, as during defaecation. She must not be disturbed by the passage of flatus. She must learn to rest during the contractions, to relax* the muscles of her hands, feet, abdomen and pelvis, to close her eyes and breathe calmly, and to avoid dissipating her energy.

The woman will be told, as is usual at this stage of labour, that she must no longer push. She is told to push again when the placenta is to be evacuated. She must be warned that a certain amount of bleeding, about 200–300 cm^3, is harmless, because during pregnancy the volume of the blood is increased. She is also told that a cold feeling and shivering can occur after delivery.

Sixth session.—This is a session devoted to synthesis. The interview stresses the joys of maternity, the comfort of the hospital, the attention of the staff, and the emotional help she will meet with during the labour. All the knowledge she has acquired during the preparation must be consolidated. She can be put into contact with women who have already gone through childbirth using the

---

*The use of the relaxation has varied. For the Russians, relaxation is accompanied by a cortical inhibition: phasic or hypnoidal states of different intensities occur, during which suggestibility is increased. In 1950, VELVOVSKI et al. [559] still used phasic states 'to obtain a reflex-conditioned consolidation of the analgesic effect of the procedures'. This technique they considered as temporary only. In the 1951 *Directions* the 'relaxing-rest' was still used for all women. In 1954 PLOTITCHER [430] recommended muscular relaxation, without speaking of hypnoidal states. As will be seen later, their use is reserved for cases needing a special approach.

method. These interviews are carried out in the doctor's presence. The woman's attention must be focused on all the details of hygiene and the examinations which will be carried out in the course of the birth, and to developing the attitude of discipline.

(iv) Mistakes during the Preparation

(1) An insufficient analysis of the history and a misunderstanding of certain problems which would have required psychotherapeutic help.

(2) Insufficient or incorrect preparation, whether in the physiotherapeutic preparation (at the expulsive phase) or in the use of language inappropriate to the intellectual level of the woman, or because of an indifferent tone of voice of the preparer.

(3) Incorrect preparation of the woman in the subjective experiences of childbirth (for instance when she is told that she will feel nothing).

(4) Lack of a 'psycho-hygienic' culture: indifference and lack of kindness and warmth amongst the staff of the maternity unit.

(v) Preparation of Women with Complications during Pregnancy and Childbirth.

Some women require an individual preparation, either partial or total (cf. the combined methods p. 129). Plotitcher classifies them into three groups:

(1) Those in whom there is a slight possibility of complications in the course of labour, for instance, women with slightly contracted pelves, herniae, or obesity. These cases require one or two supplementary sessions. The mildly anxious, also in this group, need one or two individual sessions, with a more extended psychotherapeutic contact. Sessions of 'relaxing-rest' will be used, which produce a mild inhibition (hypnoid states). In this condition 'the suggestions will be better assimilated and more firmly fixed in the women's consciousness'.

(2) Here the probability of a difficult childbirth is greater. Example: Dystocic presentation—cardiac disorder. Psychotherapy must be used here—'Action through speech, in the shape of direct suggestion in the waking state or even in hypnotic

sleep'. The woman must also be prepared for the possible use of narcotics. Hypnosis, through the mechanism of reflex conditioned inhibition, will facilitate the action of drugs in the narcosis.

(3) Emotional lability and neurotic reactions. In general, three possible reactions are seen, depending on whether the patients are hysterics, psychasthenics or neurasthenics. These patients have a 'weak' nervous system, but the determination of this type is in fact practically impossible. The study of clinical reactions alone is sufficient: a detailed history will lead to the diagnosis. These cases are given psychotherapy whilst using, in large measure, suggestion and hypnosis.

CHICHKOVA and IVANOV [91] have described a combined method for women suffering from toxaemias and cardiovascular disorders (cf. p. 130). BESKROVNAIA [44] has devoted a study to the problem of the course of childbirth in women suffering from complications during pregnancy and labour (cf. p. 145). These women need particular attention, their preparation ought to begin after the first antenatal consultation. Eventually, individual sessions will be necessary.

(b) *The Course of Labour*

CHOUGOM [93] who has studied this part of the method, believes that 'the correct organization of the work of the staff of the maternity unit constitutes the decisive and final link in the psychoprophylactic method'.

Three essential tasks confront the staff:

(1) Adequate obstetrical care;

(2) A 'psychohygienic' atmosphere;

(3) The maintenance of a good cortical tonus—that is (a) all the elements in childbirth ought to be correctly explained, (b) the pain-reducing procedures ought to be properly used and (c) the behaviour in the expulsive phase must be supervized.

(i) *Admission to the Maternity Unit*

The essential task is the creation of a good contact on admission. After taking the obstetrical history, the woman is asked some questions on the preparation. The notes recording the detailed observations on the preparation ought to go with the woman.

She is asked what has happened between the last session and her admission to the hospital, and for any traumatic events which may have occurred. If the preparation has been incomplete, it will be completed as much as is possible. A gynaecological examination is then carried out. The woman should not be allowed to mix with non-prepared women, or women with pathological pregnancies. The doctor ought to explain to the woman the important role of the midwife, and to enjoin her to follow out her instructions. He must himself ascertain whether the woman correctly applies the 'procedures'.

(ii) Conduct during the Childbirth

Care must be taken that the procedures are correctly used with regard to the particular phase of the birth. Chaotic use of procedures without supervision by the staff should be avoided because the efficacy of these procedures can be diminished if they are not used properly.* Recourse will be had from time to time to the parturient's self-control; every hour, timing herself, for several minutes she will control the length and the frequency of the contractions. If the two first procedures are sufficient, the third and fourth need not be used. The greatest attention is needed at the moment of complete dilatation. The doctor or midwife at this time can carry out the procedures instead of the woman if she is too exhausted. She should be told not to close her eyes during the contractions so as to avoid states of inhibition. It is also necessary to see that she collaborates properly in the expulsive effort. Changes in the team are very important; the doctor himself should be present when there is a change of midwife and every effort should be made not to leave the woman alone. If she has to be left alone, she must be warned, so that she knows she is alone to carry out the procedures. If the woman complains of

*As we have seen (p. 56) Goodrich gives the same advice with regard to the practice of relaxation in Read's method. In this form, relaxation is not concerned with passivity, as indeed some critics of Read's method have noted when differentiating it from the psychoprophylactic method. It would appear, moreover, to be a phenomenon of the concentration of attention, or of cortical activation in the sense in which Velvovski uses it. Its action then would be analogous to that of the 'analgesic procedures' in the psychoprophylactic method (respiration, abdominal effleurage, etc.).

pain, it should not be disregarded but she should be given something to suppress it. Advice should be given in an understanding manner which does not provoke fear. Her feeding should be watched and she should take moderate amounts of food three or four times a day. If the application of forceps turns out to be necessary, according to Chougom anaesthesia can be dispensed with in women who have been prepared, although Nicolaiev prefers anaesthesia.

(iii) Measures to be taken after the Birth and the Delivery

The genital organs will be inspected and if necessary tears will be repaired under local anaesthesia so as to avoid the pain which might possibly influence the course of a later childbirth. As the woman finds herself in a state of light inhibition, use can be made of this to give her suggestions with regard to the puerperal period. These suggestions are as follows: that she will have an urge to urinate, followed by a micturition, at the sight of the water brought for washing, some time after the delivery; that she will have a spontaneous bowel movement on the third day; that she must obey the doctor with regard to her nutrition; that she will secrete milk when the baby is put to the breast. By suggestion, the regulation of lactation will be assured.

Since 1949, Velvovski's team has used verbal suggestion to regulate lactation and has obtained satisfactory results. Their work is based on the studies of Platonov and Zdravomyslov.

(iv) Causes of Failure during the Childbirth

Agitation in women who have been prepared can be due to the following factors.

(1) *Obstetrical causes.*—In 41 per cent of failures Chougom found that the appearance of agitation in women who had been quite calm in the first phase of childbirth was the result of an obstetrical disorder such as cervical rigidity, or delayed rupture of the membranes, when dilatation is complete. These can be remedied by the artificial rupture of the membranes or by the use of drugs to relieve the cervical spasm. Under these conditions, in prolonged labours the procedures should only be used sparingly.

(2) *Chaotic use of the procedures.*—The procedures must be used carefully if they are not to lose their efficacy. The late arrival of the woman at the maternity hospital must be avoided.

(3) *Untimely stimulation of labour.*—The calm behaviour of the woman can sometimes lead to error on the part of the doctor who will be wrongly led to believe that labour is slowing up. Whenever labour is speeded up, then a verbal formula suggesting painlessness must always be added to the medication.

(4) *Incomplete psychological anamnesia.*—As a result of an incomplete anamnesis, a woman can be put into a group, when she really ought to have had an individual preparation.

(5) *Non-observation of psychohygienic rules.*—'Psycho-infection' will be avoided if women who have been prepared are not put in contact with women who have not been prepared. The non-observation of the principle of 'asepsis of behaviour and of speech' by the nursing staff must be combated; all phrases making allusions to pain, or to the possible complications of childbirth should be avoided and any attitude capable of being interpreted as unkind or indifferent should also be avoided.

The following corrections were made at the Kiev Conference to the Psychoprophylactic Method:

—The increase of the factor of suggestion. Konstantinov said on this point that the 'best results in psychoprophylaxis will be obtained by doctors who are capable of suggestion. They do not always deliberately use their power; psychoprophylactic preparation, inasmuch as it is a procedure which is used *en masse*, will be more effective if doctors can usefully link the educational and suggestive parts. For this to occur they ought to be convincing, penetrating and sure of themselves; their looks, their gestures, ought to have a favourable influence and the conversation ought to leave a strong and durable impression'. Nicolaiev also recommends the use of suggestion in all the sessions and that more attention should be paid to indirect suggestion. Jordania and Petrov-Maslakov are of the same opinion.

—Physiotherapeutic elements: Training in muscul arrelaxation according to the stage of labour (Nicolaiev), and physical training during pregnancy (Belochapko, Nicolaiev); and the greater use of medication (cf. p. 135).

(c) Extemporary Methods

The ideal would be for all women to receive complete preparation. However, for those who have not been prepared an extemporary method must be used. Its success will depend on the qualities of the staff of the maternity units as well as on the personality of the woman herself.

(i) Extemporary Psychoprophylactic Preparation

Direction 142 of the Ministry of Health of the Soviet Union recommends extemporary preparations. A good emotional contact and the suppression of fear is insisted upon, and according to the time available the procedures will be taught speedily, and the woman will be confronted with women who have gone through their childbirth successfully. If the woman has started the first stage, then the training will be carried out between the contractions. If she has entered into an advanced stage of labour, the procedures will be directly brought into use; the method to be adopted will vary according to whether completely non-prepared women are being dealt with or those who have been partially prepared. ASSATOUROV *et al.* [22] published good results obtained with this technique.

(ii) Extemporary Hypnosuggestive Preparation

KOGANOV [274], of Kharkov, uses hypnosis more than anything else in the extemporary preparation. He has published a study of 1300 cases of childbirth delivered with this method. He uses direct and indirect suggestion in the waking state and suggestion under hypnosis. In a certain number of women analgesia was obtained by means of posthypnotic suggestion with delivery in a waking state; the others were delivered under hypnosis. SIROTA [507], of Tashkent, also uses hypnosis in extemporary preparation.

(d) Combined Methods

(i) With Hypnosuggestive Procedures

As has been indicated in the discussion of theory, Zdravomyslov included elements of psychoprophylaxis in his hypnosuggestive method. The pregnancies in which Plotitcher (a member of Velvovski's team) partly uses hypnosis, have been enumerated previously. They are chiefly complicated pregnancies, either with a somatic pathology, whether obstetrical or not, or neurotic states. Platonov recommends the episodic use of the different variants of the hypnosuggestive method as an adjuvant to the psychoprophylactic method. BELOCHAPKO and FOI [38] describe the combined method of Okouniev which is carried out at the Clinic of the First Pavlov Medical Institute, Leningrad. The women follow a course of preparation from the thirty-fifth to the thirty-seventh week. The first three sessions are identical with those of the psychoprophylactic method, with the sole difference that the women are asked to carry out autosuggestion linked with respiratory exercises. After the three sessions of the psychoprophylactic method, the woman undergoes sessions of hypnotic inhibition (up to five in number), in the course of which, in a partial sleep, one tries to consolidate all that has been said in the preceding courses. It is frequently stressed moreover that the birth will be painless. Okouniev uses the figures one to three to indicate the degree of hypnosis; three is a state of deep hypnotic sleep, two a less deep state and one a light state of somnolence. He believes that the aptitude for accepting a suggestion depends on the depth attained in the course of the preparation. According to the depth, he has been able to predict the degree of pain reduction in the course of the birth. He believes that this method is helpful in cases where a positive result using the classical psychoprophylactic method is not certain.

CHICHKOVA and IVANOV [91] of Moscow have developed a method for women suffering from:

(1) Pre-eclamptic toxaemia (thirty cases), mild and severe with albuminuria, hypertension and papilloedema. The women, certain of whom were hospitalized in the department for pathological pregnancy, underwent four sessions of psychoprophylaxis. In view of the importance of the nervous system in toxaemia they were also given a course of rational psychotherapy and in severe cases underwent a hypnotic sleep.* A lowering of the blood pressure and the disappearance of albuminuria was often obtained. Twenty-five of these women went into labour spontaneously, two needed forceps delivery and three were delivered in other maternity units.

(2) Cardiovascular affections (nineteen cases) in whom a therapeutic abortion had been considered in view of the gravity of the situation. This had been put to the women but they had all refused it. In these women the preparation began very early

*Stovkis of Leyden noticed that pregnant women with mild toxaemia are more easily hypnotized than the average woman.

and they underwent 'a psychoprophylactic preparation in the form of rational psychotherapy' combined with special gymnastic exercises. Twelve went into labour spontaneously and seven had to be delivered by forceps.

NICOLAIEV [393] recommends '. . . in women of the weak and unbalanced Nervous Type and above all in the presence of difficulties with regard to the suppression of fear or when there is a lack of confidence, the carrying out of one or two sessions in the state of relaxing-rest (following Astakhov and Doniguevitch), that is to say in a state of light inhibition obtained by suggestion or, as Chichkova recommends, in a true hypnotic sleep'.

Doniguevitch carries out the technique of relaxation-rest in women who present somatic or psychological complications of their pregnancy. When the psychoprophylactic method was first used, this technique was applied to all the women, nowadays it is only used in cases where the educational effect alone is insufficient. In these cases it is important to consolidate the latter 'during the states of inhibition in which the assimilation of the teaching of the physician will be particularly effective'. He describes his technique, in which 'after each session all that has been taught is briefly formulated and consolidated by numerous repetitions with the patient in the state which has been called relaxation-rest'.

Doniguevitch is not opposed to the use of hypnotic states; he even believes that they are useful, but he tries to divest his procedure of any aura of hypnotism or of the atmosphere of mystery which usually surrounds this procedure in the public imagination. While certain authors use the common technique of hypnosis, Doniguevitch simplifies it. He avoids the use of a soft couch and the darkening of the room, authoritarian suggestions such as 'you will go to sleep, you must sleep' are replaced by words such as 'total relaxation, rest'. He also excludes from his technique 'visual fixation or counting and anything which in any way can recall the idea of hypnosis'. Doniguevitch's technique can be summed up thus; amongst his directives (dietetics, general hygiene, etc.) he recommends one hour's sleep during the day; this sleep ought always to begin at the same time and this must correspond to the time at which the next session of preparation will end. He points out that at the beginning, through lack of habit, the woman will find difficulties in going to sleep;

she should therefore remain in bed with her eyes closed, thinking of nothing, and the third or fourth time she will fall asleep. He also tells the woman that this sleep will be used to 'consolidate the new directives which have been given in the course of the session, as well as to facilitate the assimilation of the teaching which has already been given', and goes on to say 'as you know by experience, you retain particularly well what you have just repeated before going to sleep'. The doctor sees her again about five or six days later at a time which precedes her daily sleep. At the end of the session, the doctor tells the woman that the time for her usual rest has come and he invites her to sit down in an easy chair and close her eyes, to listen to him and to begin to relax. Here *in extenso* are the doctor's directives.

'In a contained, levelled and measured voice the doctor insistently repeats several times that at the time at which the woman takes her usual rest, involuntarily she will let herself be overcome by sleep, her eyelids will become heavy, a sensation of fatigue will spread over her and progressively she will enter into an agreeable state of relaxation, of rest, her breathing will become equal and deep, etc. The doctor points out that in spite of the slight sleepiness which the woman can feel on account of the habit she has developed of sleeping at this particular time, she will also distinctly hear the voice of the doctor and all his instructions. The doctor's voice will not interfere with her repose, but on the contrary, by having a calming effect on her, will calm her and plunge her deeper and deeper into a state of repose. At the same time she will be asked to concentrate all her attention on the doctor's words, without allowing herself to be distracted by any other noise or by any other thought. Ten or fifteen minutes after the end of these instructions, when the deep breathing of the woman still indicates total rest, for 10 to 15 minutes the doctor repeats, in an abbreviated form, the contents of the session, putting particular stress on the passages which demonstrate that the coming childbirth will take place without pain. Before ending the session, the doctor warns the woman that after her rest she will feel a sensation of well-being and elation just as after every rest or sleep and that in the following session this state of relaxing-rest will become more and more marked'.

After having described his method, Doniguevitch enumerates

its advantages over the classical methods of hypnosis. He considers that there is no element of surprise or of the unknown in his method: the woman understands the reflex-conditioned mechanism of going to sleep, she does not go to sleep because the doctor wants her to but because she herself has learnt the habit. Thus, thanks to the method, he avoids the mysterious aspects of hypnosis, whilst profiting from the inhibitory states in which verbal action is very effective. With regard to the much debated problem of activity-passivity, Doniguevitch considers that by his technique, he does not only obtain 'a passive progression of inhibition' (which takes place in hypnosis), but an 'active and conscious training of cortical functions and of the reflex-conditioned activity of the organism'. After one or two sessions of relaxing through 'education-activation (excitation)-prophylaxis' rest, the women see with astonishment the disappearance of heartburn, the reappearance of appetite, the improvement in their nightly sleep and in their intestinal functioning. Just as precise as are his descriptions of his technique, so his physiological explanations lack clarity and remain hypothetical; thus he admits that suggestion enters a great deal into this procedure, but sees in it the pre-eminence of reflex conditioned mechanisms. This is for two reasons, the logical connections of which are not very clear. (1) Suggestion itself 'is the most typical conditioned-reflex' (Pavlov); (2) 'suggestion in his method passes to the second level, giving first place to the active and conscious training of reflex-conditioned activity'.

It can be seen that in the Soviet Union, in spite of the scientific explanations which the Pavlovian School has put forward for hypnosis, prejudices against it may be found just as elsewhere. These prejudices probably form one of the major reasons why hypnosis has given place to educational factors and to indirect suggestion in the new psychoprophylactic method. As for the neurophysiological mechanism of the analgesia (when it is obtained), the difference between the hypnosuggestive method and the psychoprophylactic method is only quantitative. Velvovski, whilst recognizing the reality and efficacy of hypnotic analgesia wants to see in the two methods two different mechanisms, analgesia by 'hypnosis–inhibition–therapy' and analgesia through education–activation (excitation)–prophylaxis'. This way of looking at the problem has not been sufficiently proved. The majority of writers no longer insist on this point; cortical activation (excitation) and inhibition are two concomitant processes, the analgesia results from the inhibitory process.

As to the difference between the commonly used hypnosis and the method of Doniguevitch, some reserve must be maintained.

(1) Hypnosis does not necessarily involve an element of surprise and of the unknown when the subject knows in advance what is going to happen. He can even, himself, bring on a hypnotic state (autohypnosis).

(2) It is a current practice in hypnosis not to use the word 'sleep'.

(3) Authoritarian formulas have been abandoned by contemporary practitioners for many years. ZDRAVOMYSLOV [585] states for instance that he has eliminated peremptory suggestions from his hypnotic technique.

(4) Passivity would, in fact, become activity because the subject consciously lets himself fall asleep. This is possible, but it would then be necessary to allow that the same change would occur in voluntary hypnosis.

(5) It therefore seems that the only difference between hypnosis and Doniguevitch's procedure lies in the fact that he avoids the use of the word hypnosis; he is certainly right if he finds the word endangers resistances in the subject.*

(ii) With Drug-induced Analgesia

Even though the majority of workers use drugs in cases of failure, BELOCHAPKO and FOI [38] also use a combination of the psychoprophylactic method and drugs when a prolonged childbirth is foreseen. A. A. STEPANOVA [510], of Lublino, recommends a combined method for isolated maternity hospitals which have only a single midwife to carry out the preparation and to direct the childbirth. She uses different drugs in cases where, for one reason or another, the preparation has not been successful. At the beginning of dilatation if the first procedure, respiration, has had no

*Personal experiments have been carried out successfully using the technique of hypnoid relaxation in women presenting somatic or psychological complications of pregnancy (women who had been eliminated from preparation by the psychoprophylactic method). Our technique is even more divested of the classical aspects of hypnosis than that of Doniguevitch.

effect then antipyrine 0·6 g and luminal 0·1 g are used, and the first procedure is then repeated. If there is still no result, abdominal effleurage is carried out. Where this fails, abdominal friction with a chloroform lotion and irradiation with blue light is then used. When there are lumbar pains the same procedures are applied to the loins. If this fails, a lotion containing belladonna, novocaine, opium and camomile is then used. During the expulsive period, the woman is watched to see that she adopts the right position and that she collaborates in her efforts at expulsion. If this does not suffice, the nasal mucous membrane is painted with ten per cent novocaine. Of 400 cases she noted 160 had a complete analgesia, in 202 the pains were diminished and in thirty-eight only were the pains very little diminished.

VARCHAVSKAIA [548] of Leningrad has recently discussed the problem of drug analgesia in women in whom the psychoprophylactic preparation was either ineffective or very little effective— in her experience, about 25 per cent of the women. She agrees with the possibility of reinforcing the usefulness of verbal methods by pharmacological means, and compares the efficiency of different drugs. As well as the classical sedatives, sulphanilamide is also very active when used in association with pethidine.

LEVIT and RABINOVITCH [326] have also used drugs in cases where the method has failed.

After the Kiev Congress the use of drugs has been more widely adopted. Iakovlev (quoted by TEREKHOVA [523]) considers that if the Psychoprophylactic Method has not produced an analgesia, it has at least produced a favourable terrain for drug analgesia.

PETROV-MASLAKOV [413] considers that the analgesiant effect of the Psychoprophylactic Method is only obtained in women of a particular personality type. He considers that some obstetricians have been disappointed in the method because of theoretical errors. Too much importance has been attached to reflex-conditioned pain. For instance, these practitioners have given up the use of drugs which might have actually produced an analgesia. Petrov-Maslakov recommends drugs for women who have not been prepared and for women who have been prepared but show signs of restlessness (a mixture of bromide, pyramidon and caffeine). This produces both a pharmacological and a suggestive action. NICOLAIEV [393] recommends drugs for women who have been prepared where there is difficulty or a complete failure, and as a preventative measure he even recommends a spasmolytic for all primiparae. In women of a weak Nervous Type the use of drugs should be systematic, such as injections directly into the cervix. Lourie believes that the combination of the psychoprophylactic method with narcotics seems to settle once and for all the problem of obstetrical analgesia.

(e) Study of the Nervous Type of Pregnant Woman

As has been seen, the study of the Nervous Type which is made by Velvovski and his team in the first session goes no further than a psychological anamnesis based on biographical data. Nicolaiev and his school have tried to elaborate a more precise method but even so it is still very approximate. Apart from the strength, the lability and the character of the relations between excitation and inhibition, these writers have tried to take into consideration certain peculiarities in the relationships between the first and the second signalling systems and between the cortex and the subcortical region.

ASTAKHOV and BESKROVNAIA [23], pupils of Nicolaiev, have elaborated the following method which is based on:

(1) a detailed case-history,

(2) observation of behaviour during the preparation and during the childbirth,

(3) a study of suggestibility,

(4) a study of the relationships between inhibition and excitation in the word-association test (Gakkel), and

(5) a plethysmographic study.

In order to compare the personality studies made in western countries with the anamnesis made in Russia, the latter will be discussed in detail.

(i) *Case History*

This consists of a detailed inquiry bearing on the following points:

The social milieu in which the woman was brought up.

Her relationships with her parents, her family and her friends.

Her behaviour at school.

Her professional activities; her professional beginnings, her capacity for work.

Her capacity for adaptation; her response to new tasks and to new environments.

Her relationships with her husband, her in-laws and his friends.

Her attitude toward children in general, toward her own children and toward the pregnancy.

Particular attention should be paid to the following points: (1) her capacity for work; (2) her perseverance; (3) her spirit of initiative; (4) her capacity for learning; (5) her interest in social questions; (6) her capacity for concentration; (7) her adaptation to new tasks; (8) her mastery of herself; (9) attitudes in the face of danger; (10) intellectual capacity; (11) adaptation to new environments; (12) her communicability; (13) her sensitivity; (14) preoccupation with her health; (15) her way of discussing her symptoms; (16) her cleanliness; (17) her calmness; (18) her capacity for attention; (19) her irritability; (20) her capacity for distraction; (21) disquietude, impatience, restlessness; (22) importunity; (23) the speed of going to sleep and waking up. This information is extremely subjective, but parents, friends and others are also seen in order to complete the information, often using a social worker.

(ii) Observation of Behaviour during the Preparation and the Childbirth

This is carried out with the help of the staff of the maternity unit.

(iii) The Study of Suggestibility (Relationships between the First and Second Signalling systems)

Several tests are used based on the works of Birman which use hypnotizability as a criterion of the Nervous Type: (1) the eyelid test of Astakhov. The eyeballs are lightly pressed upon for several seconds and suggestions are made to the woman that she will have difficulty in opening her eyes; (2) Nicolaiev's test (first described in 1927) which is similar to the 'body-sway-test'.

(iv) The Study of the Relationships between Inhibition and Excitation

Here Gakkel's word-association test (which is a technique similar to Jung's word-association tests) is given, and an attempt is made to distinguish between delayed responses which are due to inhibition and those which are due to inertia in the system of activation.

(v) *The Plethysmograph is used to Study Changes in the Blood Vessels*

JORDANIA [255] presented a paper to the Kiev conference in which he described another way in which to determine the particular Types of the women (Table 1, pp. 139–40).

LEVIT and RABINOVITCH [326] attempted to study the Nervous Type on material from the history and from the observation of the woman's behaviour. They stress that their method is incomplete owing to the subjective character of the details obtained in the questioning of the patient. The results give more information on the emotional substratum of the woman than on her particular typology. Of 1266 women prepared by the Psychoprophylactic Method they found that 526 were of a strong and balanced Nervous Type; 445 were of a strong but unbalanced Nervous Type; 121 were of a strong, balanced but inert Nervous Type, and 161 were of a weak, suggestible and unbalanced Nervous Type. They tried to predict the behaviour of the woman as well as the efficacy of the method by taking into account the general condition of the woman, the obstetrical history, the neurological examination, the supposed Nervous Type and the number of sessions which had been carried through. Notes were made on two occasions, the end of the preparation and after the delivery. The results were as follows: 'excellent' results were predicted for 656 women (51·8 per cent); 'good' for 424 women (33·4 per cent); 'mediocre' for 164 (12·9 per cent); and 'none' for 22 (1·9 per cent). The details noted in the Maternity Hospital were as follows: 'excellent' 546 (43·2 per cent); 'good' 412 (32·6 per cent); 'mediocre' 197 (19·6 per cent); 'none' 35 (2·7 per cent). Negative results were found in women of weak and unbalanced Nervous Types.

5. RESULTS

Results Concerning Analgesia and Behaviour

At the Leningrad Congress (1951), all the participants concentrated on the problem of objective criteria of pain and analgesia. In fact, no method yet exists of measuring these two phenomena. BELOCHAPKO and FOI [38] reported that Velvovski obtained positive results in 90 per cent of his cases, Nicolaiev in 85 per cent of his cases and at the Pavlov Institute in Leningrad in 75 per cent, stressed the difficulties and declared that 'the evaluation of the positive results of the Psychoprophylactic Method is greatly exaggerated, and this is explained by the fact that we do not possess objective means of measuring the pain of childbirth'. Assessments which are based on the behaviour of the woman as judged by the observer, and on the statements of the woman are not, in fact, objective. All the statistical analyses cannot be given here. In general, the evaluation of the Method is made by using a five-point scale:

'5' represents the maximum success; no pain, the parturient being conscious and active throughout the whole labour;

'4', complaints of short duration with endurable pains;

'3', failure in spite of a temporary analgesia. Three is considered by some writers as a failure, others consider it as a partial success.

'2' and '1' represent complete failure.

The following table shows the results obtained by the originators of the Method in 1200 cases at the Maternity Centre of the Central Neuro-Psychiatric Hospital of the Ministry of Transportation at Kharkov [558].

5	4	3	2 and 1
43·8 per cent	37·2 per cent	13·5 per cent	5·5 per cent

A more recent statistical analysis was published by ARNOLDOVA [20], of Astrakhan. The author analysed 571 cases prepared by the Psychoprophylactic Method and an equal number of controls. She herself prepared and delivered 71 women. She had 92 per cent of good results (54) in her personal cases, and 89 per cent in the other 500. She explains the difference as due to the fact that in her personal series, the same doctor carried out both preparations and delivery. The results were as good in aged primiparae as in young primiparae: 79 out of 106 (74 per cent) had results noted four and five. Previous complicated deliveries did not influence the results in prepared women, as opposed to what happened with the non-prepared ones. Abortions, dysmenorrhea and various gynaecological affections in the past history of the parturient women had an unfavourable effect on delivery in all the women.

Table 1. Clinical Typological Classification of Higher Nervous Activity (Jordania)

	Strong, unbalanced (excitable)	Strong, balanced (lively)	Strong, balanced (inert)	Weak, unbalanced (inhibited)
A. Basic processes of Higher Nervous Activity: 1. Excitation. 2. Inhibition.	Excitation prevails over inhibition.	The two fundamental processes occur in equal proportions.		Inhibition prevails over excitation.
B. Fundamental properties of nervous processes. 1. Force.	Satisfactory capacity for work.	Good capacity for work		Rapid tiring whilst working; submits easily; lack of perseverance.
2. Equilibrium.	Perseverance in attaining a goal. Lack of self-control; no patience; excessive behaviour reactions; lack of movements and gestures.			
3. Mobility.	Rapid transition from a state of rest to excitation.		Slow adjustment to the environment, particularly new ones; slow actions.	Indifference to outside events.
C. The state of Higher Nervous Activity at different times of life. 1. Initial period (first memories).	Takes part in and leads noisy games; wants to lead. Initiators.	Lively participation in the events of childhood.	Moderate participation in all life happenings.	Tendency to remain outside noisy games. Whining. Unwarranted sensitivity; whining; easily influenced by friends.

2. Period of sexual maturation.	Tendency to break away from parental protections.	Self-mastery in familial and daily relations.	Ill-defined manifestations of failure of ovarian function.
3. Period of sexual maturity. 4. Menopause.	Rapid manifestation of the failure of ovarian function.	Good tolerance of the failure of ovarian function.	
D. At different times in life. 1. Capacity for work and reserve of strength.	Initiative; great perseverance in attaining a goal.	Hard worker; large energy reserve.	Frequent refusal to do extra work; lack of initiative.
2. Behaviour in the face of danger.	Perseverance in overcoming obstacles.	Rapid assessment of a situation before acting.	No perseverance; tends to avoid decisions in vital situations.
3. Behaviour in a medical establishment.	Conflicts with staff; refusal of treatment.	Slow assessment of a situation before taking a decision. Complete confidence in all exigencies in hospital.	Excessive fears preceding choice of treatment.
Alcohol.	Rapid excitation.	Moderate excitation.	Debilitating effect, with weakness of the two processes.
Ether. Bromides.	Slow in going to sleep. Momentary balance of fundamental nervous processes.	Rapid sleep.	Oppression of the nervous state.
Caffeine.	Excitation increased.		When the dose is diminished, excitatory functions increase.

BESKROVNAIA [44] has obtained better results with the Psychoprophylactic Method (using 500 cases) than with a drug-induced analgesia (using 400 cases) in women presenting pathological complications, either during the pregnancy or during the childbirth; there were 33·2 per cent of failures with the Psychoprophylactic Method and 47·3 per cent of failures with the pharmocological method.

ASSATOUROV et al. [22] published an analysis of 571 deliveries made in three provincial Maternity Units. Some of these women had undergone a complete psychoprophylactic training and others an extemporary training (some had remained for several days in the hospital itself). These authors insist that the keystone of the method is a kindly atmosphere in the maternity unit. They claim to have been successful in making their staff observe all the rules of 'asepsis speech and behaviour'. Under these conditions they were able to obtain positive results in 80 per cent of cases with extemporary psychoprophylactic preparation. The results in women who had been completely prepared by the Psychoprophylactic Method rose to 91 per cent. Contrary to the general consensus of opinion the good results were just as numerous in multiparae as in primiparae.

M. SIROTA [507], of Tashkent, has presented a comparative statistical study of the efficacy of the different methods; complete Psychoprophylactic Method (58 cases), partial Psychoprophylactic Method (two sessions) (90 cases), and the method of verbal suggestion (229 cases) used when the woman arrived at the Maternity Centre. The percentage of failures was 10 per cent for the complete method, 16 per cent for the partial method and 6 per cent for the verbal suggestion method. In the case of the partial method the author lays particular stress on the time factor, and particularly on the importance of the interval between the last session and the childbirth itself. He believes that this interval ought not to exceed a fortnight in any case. Furthermore an extra session must be arranged when the woman arrives at the hospital. If this delay exceeds three weeks, the supplementary interview when the woman is admitted to the hospital may not be enough, and the conditioned reflex which has been already produced has probably disappeared. Where the preparation has been complete there is no need for an extra session.

TEREKHOVA [522], the chief obstetrician to the Ministry of Health in the Soviet Union comments at the Kiev Conference on the different results in the different regions of the country. Thus complete success varies from 14 to 69 per cent, partial success from 25 to 61 per cent, and failures from 0·5 to 31 per cent.

F. E. VARCHAVSKAIA [548] stresses the divergencies which exist between the different workers with regard to the question of failure. The proportion of cases where the analgesia was insufficient, varied from 13 to 37 per cent. She considers that these different views are due to the absence of sufficiently objective criteria for evaluating the method. She herself recorded observations on 1567 women, of whom 448 were delivered with the method of verbal analgesia, 819 with pharmacological analgesia and 300 without any analgesia at all (using this as a control group). In the first group the number of good results was 76·6 per cent; the other results in the same group were mediocre or failures. When there are good results, Varchavskaia adds, the behaviour is often found to be 'disciplined and organized' rather than a true analgesia.

From 1955 onwards a tendency has been noticed to no longer use the term 'painless childbirth' or the 'psychoprophylaxis of the pain of childbirth' but to replace it by the phrase 'psychoprophylactic preparation of pregnant women for childbirth'. The question was settled at the Kiev Congress [100] where this latter expression was adopted. Those in favour of the change brought up several arguments in its favour:

(1) The percentage of deliveries carried out by the Psychoprophylactic Method which are really painless is low. It is more often the case of a reduction in the pain and above all of a disciplining action on behaviour;

(2) By stating that the fundamental objective of the method is the suppression of pain, one runs the risk of bringing discredit on it, as this objective is not always, in fact, obtained.

(3) In fact, about 1953 [255, 334] a certain dissatisfaction was coming to be felt with regard to the method. This was not entirely due to the reason given above but was also the result of a faulty use of the method and to wrong theoretical constructions which considered that pain was a simple reflex-conditioned product.

144 PSYCHOSOMATIC METHODS IN PAINLESS CHILDBIRTH

This explains why a new title was necessary which would reflect the different aspects of the whole method.

At the Kiev Conference, Nikolaiev was the only one to defend the old title. From 1955 onwards he had believed that the title 'psychoprophylactic preparation for childbirth' was too vague. At Kiev he explained his position as follows. 'The principal task of the psychoprophylactic system is to fight against the pain of childbirth, to fight a battle for its prevention—or as it is possible to say this now—for its diminution'. He believes that the phrases 'painless', 'prophylaxis of pains' or 'pain-killing' give confidence to the woman.

Certain figures given at the Kiev Conference took separate account of the factors of analgesia and of behaviour. For instance, Belochapko and Beskrovnaia reported the statistics in the Table below (a comparative study of the results obtained in women prepared by the Psychoprophylactic Method), the values are percentages:

	Behaviour				Analgesia			
Parturients	5	4	3	2	5	4	3	2
Primiparae	60·7	28·1	8·6	2·6	15·4	44·0	30·6	10·0
Multiparae	60·0	33·0	6·0	1·0	16·0	48·0	32·5	3·5
Total	60·4	30·0	7·6	2·0	15·6	45·6	31·4	7·4

Jordania also reported that the analgesic effect was half as great as the effect on behaviour. Out of 302 women prepared by the psychoprophylactic method for at least four sessions the results were as follows (percentages):

	Complete success	Partial success	Failure
	per cent	per cent	per cent
Behaviour	79·1	12·6	8·3
Analgesia	31·7	5·5	15·2

Jordania also attempted to improve the criteria of analgesia. He presented a scheme for assessing the intensity of the pains of childbirth. He distinguished three degrees of pain:

(1) A strong pain (failure) characterized by one or more of the following signs: (a) frequent cries during the contractions, (b) motor agitation, (c) grinding of the teeth, or (d) tears during the contraction.

(2) Middling pains characterized by one or more of the following signs: (a) moaning during the delivery, (b) weak and infrequent crying, or (c) an expression of suffering.

Strong pain occurred when one of the signs of middling pain was associated with two at least of the following symptoms:

(i) pupiliary dilatation during the contraction,
(ii) acceleration of the pulse and of breathing,
(iii) oliguria,
(iv) hyperaemia of the abdominal skin, and
(v) increase in the systolic blood pressure by more than 10 mm Hg.

(3) Weak pains when all the preceding signs are absent and there are only very infrequent and slight groans.

Medical and Obstetrical Advantages

CHOUGOM [93] put forward figures showing a reduction in the average duration of labour by two hours in women who had been prepared by the Psychoprophylactic Method. He also mentioned that the number of forceps applications was diminished. Labour proceeded better in women with a contracted pelvis who had been prepared by the Psychoprophylactic method owing to their good mental equilibrium. There was also a favourable influence on the general complications of pregnancy, a diminution of the number of cases of asphyxia of the new-born, and a good influence on the puerperal period. BESKROVNAIA [44] studied the problem of the course of pathological labours in women who had been prepared by the method. She made a comparative study of three groups of women who showed complications, due either to general disturbances of pregnancy or to pathological disorders which had been present before the pregnancy, or again to dystocias of all types.

The first group submitted to psychoprophylactic preparation

comprised 500 women; the second group, who received a pharmacological analgesia, comprised 400 women; the third group, also of 400 women did not receive any analgesia.

The following results were noted by Beskrovnaia concerning the course of the labour and the puerperium.

(1) Reduction in the length of labour by two hours in the primiparae of group one as compared with primiparae of group two.

(2) The same reduction in the multiparae of group one as compared with the multiparae of the two other groups.

(3) She also noticed a very slight diminution in the number of cases of eclampsia, in group one (three cases) compared with group two (five cases) and group three (four cases).

(4) There were forty-two cases (8·4 per cent) of uterine inertia in group one, fifty-seven cases (14·2 per cent) in group two, and fifty cases (12·5 per cent) in group three.

(5) The number of forceps applications which were necessary was slightly diminished in group one, 8·6 instead of 12·7 per cent in group two and 10·5 per cent in group three.

(6) Episiotomy: group one, 19·6 per cent; group two, 32 per cent; group three, 27 per cent.

(7) Apparent death of the child: group one, 3 per cent; group two, 5·7 per cent; group three, 4·7 per cent.

(8) Stillbirths: group one, 0·6 per cent; group two, 2·1 per cent; group three, 2·1 per cent.

F. E. VARCHAVSKAIA [548] found that in women who had been delivered with verbal analgesia, the mean duration of labour was diminished by an hour and a quarter compared with women who had been deprived of all analgesia. In women who had had a pharmacological analgesia the length of labour was definitely longer than in the two other categories. The Vice-Minister of Health of the Soviet Union, CHOUPIK [94], gives comparative statistics on the pathology of pregnancy and childbirth which has been recently reported in the ten Maternity Hospitals in the Moscow Region. In women who had had the Psychoprophylactic Method the late onset toxaemias were 3·65 per cent and in other women 6·8 per cent. Stimulation of the uterus had been carried out in 4·6 per cent of the first group and 6·2 per cent in the second group. The natal mortality was 0·7 per cent in the first group and 1·7 per cent in the second group.

BELOCHAPKO [37] analysing 4000 cases of women who had been prepared by the Psychoprophylactic Method mentions that uterine inertia was found in 5·4 per cent, the natal mortality was 0·2 per cent, apparent death 1·8 per cent, death within 48 hours 0·14 per cent, and on the following day 0·17 per cent. He also made a comparative study of three groups of women, 500 who had been prepared by the Psychoprophylactic Method, 400 by pharmacological analgesia and 400 who had not received any analgesia. The proportions of complications of pregnancy and of labour in the three groups were lowest in the first and highest in the second.

ARNOLDOVA [20], noted a decrease in the duration of the period of dilatation: 10 hours 53 minutes in prepared women instead of 17 hours 50 minutes for the non-prepared (the study covered 500 women in each group). In addition, all women had a feeling of well-being at the end of the preparation. Out of 571 women, 92 had toxaemic disorders, with edema in 85, and nephropathy in seven. In the control group, 124 were affected with toxaemia, with edema in 112, nephropathy in eleven and eclampsia in one. A comparison of the two groups showed, in prepared women, four cases of bleeding due to uterine inerti (13 in controls) eight cases of foetal distress (26 in controls), nineteen cases of uterine inertia (201 in controls), 66 untimely ruptures of the membranes (192 in controls), 7·8 per cent perineal lacerations (14·4 per cent in controls), 17·6 per cent of rupture of the cervix (20·4 per cent in controls), 38 cases of local puerperal disorders (104 in controls), 13 cases of foetal anoxia (27 in controls), four cases of still-birth (seven in controls), and a neo-natal death (four in controls). Forceps were used in 12 prepared women and in 31 women of the control group; episiotomy was performed in 35 prepared women and 52 controls, and manual delivery in three and nine cases respectively. An increase in bodyweight when leaving the maternity hospital was found in 419 infants of prepared women against 354 infants of non-prepared mothers.

As to the total number of women who have been delivered using the Psychoprophylactic Method precise statistics are not available. In 1953 it was estimated that the number was 300,000.* TEREKHOVA [523] reports that in Russia obstetrical analgesia by the Psychoprophylactic Method or the pharmacological method has changed from 17·7 per cent in the towns in 1949 to 55·6 per cent in 1954, and in the country the figure rose from 3·6 per cent to 36·7 per cent. The method has spread from the Soviet Union to several other countries. In China† (100,000 deliveries carried out in 1955) [132], in Poland [324, 514], in Czechoslovakia [74, 220, 233, 234, 566, 567], in Bulgaria [130], in East Germany and in France, whence the method has spread to other countries in Europe and America.

6. PSYCHOPHYSIOLOGICAL STUDIES

Psychophysiological studies concerning the psychoprophylaxis of the pain of childbirth are still rudimentary. They have been carried out with a view to objectivizing the results of the Psychoprophylactic Method. The plethysmograph has been used to study vascular reactions. JELOKHOVTSEVA [251] and KHETCHINACHVILI [264] have shown that verbal action through hypnosis or through the Psychoprophylactic Method was able to influence the plethysmographic tracings. Disturbed tracings brought about by fear or by traumatic words became regular again after the psychoprophylactic preparation.

Velvovski reports that NIKOULINE [395] has studied one hundred cases and found that the amount of blood adrenaline was half as much in women delivered by the Psychoprophylactic Method as in women who had not been prepared. The presence of acetylcholine,

*We have taken this figure from VERMOREL [561] where it is given without a reference. At the Kiev Conference figures for the whole of the Soviet Union wee not produced. SYROVATKO [519], 1957, speaks of the millions of women who have been prepared for childbirth by the Psychoprophylactic Method.

†HELLMAN [227], a German obstetrician who had spent several years in China before World War II, considers that childbirth is easier in that country on account of the woman's attitude toward it. She considers the birth of a child as a gain, which betters her position in the family. Delivery is already more difficult in women who have lived abroad as students.

which is found in the blood of women during painful contractions, was not discovered by Nikouline in women who had been prepared, and Velvovski was able to confirm these results himself.

SYROVATKO and IAKHONTOV [518] reported on the E.E.G.s of nine women taken during their pregnancy and in different stages of delivery; three deliveries took place with pharmacological analgesia, six of the women benefited from a psychoprophylactic preparation, either complete or extemporary. They found that psychoprophylactic preparation produced calm behaviour during the delivery and this was reflected in the E.E.G. The changes in the alpha rhythm during the contractions were minimal, both in the women who had had a complete preparation and in those who had had only an extemporary preparation. Syrovatko and Yakhontov write 'verbal action via the second signalling system modifies the functioning of the cerebral cortex of the parturient as is shown in the modifications of the E.E.G. tracings'. They put forward a physiological interpretation of the mechanisms underlying the analgesias, believing that a strong contraction leads to a cortical excitation, which then spreads. Drug action inhibits this excitation whilst verbal action limits its diffusion. They believe that the electroencephalogram cannot explain the physiological mechanism of childbirth but can help to clarify certain phenomena at work in the analgesia. TEREKHOVA [523] at the Kiev Conference mentions amongst others the researches of IAKOVLEV et al. [239] of Sverdlovsk who studied the cortical electrical activity of women who had undergone the Psychoprophylactic Method, and BOULAVINTSEVA [56] of Leningrad was able to demonstrate, using the oxyhaemoglobimeter, that the method had a favourable effect on the oxygen level of the arterial blood.

ARNOLDOVA [20], in the above mentioned study, reported physiological data about the feeling of pain. She investigated uterine contractions by the method of external hysterography, and studied a group of 142 women, half of whom had been prepared. She analysed 425 tracings: the duration of the period of dilatation depends on the rhythm of uterine activity, i.e. on the regularity of contractions and the intervals between them. The interval in prepared women was two to three minutes, the duration of contraction 60–70 seconds. In non-prepared women, the intervals were unequal and the duration of contractions 40–50 seconds. Thus, out of 236 recorded tracings in non-prepared women, 120 showed irregular intervals and 63 contractions of variable duration. But out of 189 tracings recorded in prepared women, only 15 showed non-rhythmic intervals and six a variable duration of contraction.

Arnoldova also studied the reaction to pain plethysmographically. Fifty-nine recordings were made, 29 from 16 prepared parturient women, and 30 from an equal number of controls. In the prepared women, the author recorded eight regular tracings corresponding to painless childbirth. Fifteen tracings showed a flattening in women who had experienced an unpleasant feeling, and tension in the lower abdomen during contractions. A flattening was also noted in two tracings of women who had pains, but not during contractions. Two tracings showed respiratory oscillations during contractions. One tracing showed an increase in amplitude in a parturient woman who had felt a sensation of warmth and had presented cutaneous hyperemia. In a woman whose delivery had been classified as a failure, the tracing showed a flattening during contraction. Among non-prepared women, two women had a painless childbirth with a regular tracing; of 14 women whose deliveries had been painful, flattening of the curve was noted in 19 recordings; four tracings showed respiratory oscillations, four showed an increased amplitude simultaneously with the subjective feeling of pain (with sweating and redness of the skin). In conclusion, the author considered that the plethysmographic tracing was stable in prepared women. A mild flattening was associated with the unpleasant feeling whereas in non-prepared women, the flattening which corresponded to pain was more marked. Arnoldova also studied changes in the blood count of parturient women, and considered that strong pains induce leukocytosis. She also noted an increase in blood pressure during delivery in 15 prepared women (out of 71) and in 56 non-prepared ones (out of 71). Lastly, a strong pain during childbirth may result in the release of ketone in the urine. She found this ketonuria during complete dilatation in eight of the 71 prepared women and in 32 per cent of the 71 non-prepared.

CHAPTER 10

THE APPLICATION OF THE PSYCHOPROPHYLACTIC METHOD IN FRANCE AND THROUGHOUT THE WORLD

THE Psychoprophylactic Method has been practised by Lamaze and Vellay at the Polyclinique des Métallurgistes in Paris, since 1952. Several other maternity Units have followed their example both in Paris and in provincial towns. It was following a trip to Russia in 1951 that Lamaze, impressed by the results that he had witnessed there, undertook to introduce the Psychoprophylactic Method into France. In 1954 he was able to reaffirm his decision 'of following and spreading more widely a work which was undertaken with faith and enthusiasm, for but one aim, which appears to be nothing less than the fundamental transformation of the status of women in the world'. Lamaze has devoted himself to this cause with an ardour equal to that of his English colleague, Grantly Dick Read. But he was not exposed to the same indifference as the latter. Theoretical controversies arose—some reservations were felt—but on the whole the interest of the method was recognized. So it was that the Municipal Council of Paris in April 1954 voted funds for experiments in the method to be made in different Maternity Units in the city.

The application of the method was the object of a detailed description in the *Revue de la Nouvelle Médecine* (special number— May 1954), in the thesis of H. Vermorel, *L'Accouchement sans douleur*, and in a work for a larger public which came from Lamaze and his team [297]. A study devoted entirely to technique appeared under the signatures of M. and A. BOURREL and COLETTE JEANSON [58]. Numerous other publications were devoted to the method, such as those by LAMAZE and his collaborators [293–306], VELLAY [551, 552], ANGELERGUES [15–18], and BOURREL [57, 58]. The work of other writers will be considered at the end of this chapter. An important report was also made by LAMAZE to the International Congress of Gynaecology and Obstetrics in Havana (December 1955) [296]. Another more recent communication is that of Lamaze and Vellay given at the meeting in Paris on 7 April 1957 [303].

These different publications, as well as the description that we have already given of the Soviet method, give details of the French method, which is directly derived from the Russian one. It will be sufficient to mention the practical modifications that have occurred and to consider several problems which have arisen from the theoretical point of view.

The details of the practical application of the method refer to the technique used at the Polyclinique des Métallurgistes. The modifications of this technique, as used by other units will be mentioned later.

NOMENCLATURE

The French practitioners preserve the title of Painless Childbirth, in spite of the terminological modifications recommended at the Kiev Conference. Their position approaches that of Nicolaiev who, during the Congress, put forward a plea in favour of keeping to the old title.

The reasons advanced by VELLAY [552] lack precision. It seems that he is chiefly concerned with the prestige of the expression 'Painless Childbirth', which has a powerful effect on women. ECONOMIDES and VERMOREL [143] more explicitly state 'that this nomenclature is useful in the sense that painless childbirth is a possibility in a sufficient number of cases, and that psychoprophylaxis envisages this possibility for the future on a large scale'. They attribute, moreover, 'An undeniable therapeutic value' to this expression.

THE NUMBER OF SESSIONS

The preparation comprises nine sessions. The number is reduced in certain maternity units; six sessions may be enough. In contradistinction to the practice in the Soviet Union, where the first session is considered to be of exceptional importance, and is entirely individual, in France all the sessions are group sessions, ten to twelve pregnant women making up the group. The women are not selected with regard to education. The last study by LAMAZE [297] recommended eight sessions. That of BOURREL et al. [58] seven, plus a preliminary course for husbands.

PERSONNEL

French practitioners have introduced an innovation by entrusting six sessions to a physiotherapist. The theoretical courses are given by an obstetrician and a psychiatrist (Bourrel considers that the latter is not necessary) gives a lecture on the physiology of the nervous system. In certain maternity units the responsibility for the preparation is entrusted to a doctor who has specialized in this field, either an obstetrician or a psychiatrist. This doctor is sometimes assisted by a physiotherapist, sometimes by a midwife. The preparation may be left on occasion to the midwife.

THE SESSIONS

According to BOURREL et al. [58] whose recent work contains the most detailed description of the preparation, this involves a preliminary session for husbands and seven sessions for the women. Each comprises a theoretical part followed by exercises consisting, according to the stage of the preparation, of respiratory exercises, muscular relaxation and training in the positions for delivery. The authors do not recommend gymnastic exercises, in particular proscribing those which bring the abdominal muscles too violently into play. They only recommend movements of the feet and legs aiming to loosen up the joints.*

The first session deals with fertilization and the physiology of the first three months of pregnancy.

The second session deals with the period of pregnancy lasting from the fourth month to term. The importance of the nervous system is explained and the development of the foetus is demonstrated.

The third session deals with the principle of the method—the suppression of fear—and gives a long explanation of reflexology. The woman's activity is continually stressed, she is told that no attempt will be made to *distract* her at the time of childbirth but on the contrary to *integrate* her with her delivery and to make her fully aware of the contractions. The rational factor and the understanding acquired by the woman which raise the level of consciousness are ceaselessly stressed.

The fourth session deals with the role of respiration; it provides

*As we have seen NICOLAIEV (1956) returns to a greater use of gymnastics (p. 128) in the preparation.

a good oxygen supply and also trains the abdominal and diaphragmatic muscles.

The fifth session deals with neuromuscular education, an active phenomenon which ought to maintain and raise the threshold of sensibility of the brain. It is practically similar to the technique of progressive relaxation used by Read.

The sixth session deals with the physiological phenomena of dilatation and of the behaviour which the woman ought to adopt. From the phase of a three-finger dilatation on, the woman will use shallow and fast breathing with simultaneous muscular release. Between the contractions she will relax so as to conserve her maximum strength.

The seventh session gives a physiological explanation of delivery, and the posture which should be adopted in this phase is demonstrated.

In comparison the theoretical content of the Russian preparation is much simpler. For instance, according to PLOTITCHER [430], the reflexological explanations are reserved for more sophisticated women. KIRITCHENKO's brochure [266] does not mention them at all.

The interpretation of the mode of action of the different exercises varies a great deal. For instance, the Soviet writers allow that the exercises, chiefly respiratory, produce a distraction during contractions.

It is true that French writers have wished to adapt the method to French women, but considering the complexity of their explanations, it could be asked whether they had not overestimated the intellectual capacities of their audience. As described by these authors, the content of these sessions appears too important, and the level too high, although from what we have observed in practice this theoretical approach is undoubtedly made easier by some instructors. According to BOURREL the atmosphere in which the sessions are held is important—it ought to be charged with confidence. 'This confidence is serious, reflective, rational, just as much as the training itself is serious, reflective and rational'.

It can be seen that Bourrel tries to avoid all emotional elements in the relationship between the doctor and the woman he is preparing. Their conversation should be essentially a means of education, and ought never to consist of 'free emotional discharge in an atmosphere of Spiritism' (ANGELERGUES [15]). These writers seem to employ an excessively rigorous attitude, at least, theoretically. It must be said that in those sessions which we have attended in various maternity units, some of which were being carried out by skilled psychotherapists, a good emotional atmosphere was the rule. The Russians themselves have recommended this, indeed they use the first individual session primarily to create a good relationship.

The doctor in charge of the preparation ought to be able to answer all the questions which are put to him. According to Bourrel, one of the inevitable questions is this, 'Why do midwives and women doctors suffer in childbirth?' These women, knowing all that is desirable about childbirth surely ought not to suffer. 'The reply is very simple,' Bourrel writes, at once pointing out that it is due to the non-Pavlovian outlook of the women in question. However, at the Kiev Conference, Konstantinov quoted the personal experiences of women doctors and midwives in Russia, probably trained on Pavlovian lines, who suffer just as much as other women. On this account he considered that the didactic element alone is insufficient to produce an analgesia, and stressed his view that the psychotherapeutic element (suggestion) was equally as important [277].

EXERCISES

The respiratory technique is different to that which is carried out in Russia. The majority of workers use rapid superficial respiration (formerly called panting respiration).* Some consider that it tires the woman and use the respiratory exercises recommended by the Russians (BAUX and FERRIER [33]).

In place of the original psychoprophylactic practice of 'relaxing-rest' which has as its aim a 'reflex-conditioned consolidation' of the verbal action on the pregnant woman, Lamaze and his followers introduced a technique of neuromuscular education, very similar to that practised by Read.

*The mode of action of this type of respiration is controversial. It is claimed to improve oxygenation, but it is possible that this rapid respiration induces hypercapnia, with an analgesiant effect, at the same time producing a diversion of attention, or in Pavlovian terms, a centre of cortical excitation. (See Note, p. 16).

THEORY

The theoretical aspects of the method have been developed chiefly by Lamaze, Angelergues and Vermorel. Founded on Pavlovian principles, which have already been described in the discussion on the Soviet methods, in some respects Lamaze and Angelergues do not take into account the divergences of opinion which were manifested in Russia at the Leningrad Congress of 1951. Vermorel mentions them but does not consider them in as much detail as one would like. For instance Lamaze and Angelergues hold to the original views of Velvovski, assigning a purely reflex-conditioned origin to the pain of childbirth. They do not take the unconditional factor sufficiently into account, the importance of which was stressed at the Kiev Conference in 1956. Vermorel cites the several viewpoints that exist in Russia concerning the genesis of the pain of childbirth, and the modifications that Velvovski has had to make to his original conceptions. Nevertheless in his 1955 report LAMAZE [296] mentions only emotional and reflex-conditioned factors.

In 1957 ANGELERGUES and ROELENS [17] have a less dogmatic attitude. 'Many studies', they write, 'will yet be necessary to clarify the mystery of pain in childbirth'. But they still emphasize the conditioned reflex origin of this pain: 'not a simple conditioned reflex, but a complex organization of groups of conditioned reflexes, of dynamic stereo-types'. However, 'it does not mean that the conditional determination of pain is exclusively verbal: other elements play a role, although of a second order'. On the other hand Lamaze and Angelergues seem to agree with Velvovski on the two mechanisms of analgesia: the one by excitation which leads to an increase of the threshold of the pain (prophylaxis); the other by inhibition (or therapy). In their account they envisage above all 'the active state of the cortex', 'cortical activation', etc., and reject the factor of inhibition.*

The position Vermorel takes up is not so definite. He appears to admit the positive role of inhibition in certain conditions, but his interpretation lacks clarity. Thus, the aim of the respiratory exercises is, he said, 'to produce a powerful cortical focus, capable

---

*This is a theory which was disputed at the Leningrad Congress and abandoned at the Kiev Congress by the majority of Soviet workers. Inhibition is considered as the primordial factor in analgesia [131].

of inhibiting the uterine impulses which are coming up to the cortex'. He also writes, 'The procedures of analgesia which the woman is taught . . . constitute the means of creating foci of activity which will inhibit the conditional and unconditional painful reflexes'. But he does not state whether he considers, as does Velvovski, that a process of excitation produces an elevation of the cortical threshold to pain or whether it is a mechanism of inhibition which is in operation, as in the procedures of indirect suggestion. It is otherwise difficult to solve this problem because the two processes of excitation and of inhibition are complementary and inseparable. This duality, introduced by Velvovski, seems likely not to be shown in the present state of our knowledge of the central formation of pain sensation.

Velvovski's theory was already contested at the Congress of Leningrad (1951). After the Kiev Congress (1956) it is abandoned by most Soviet authors. Inhibition is considered as the primary factor in analgesia [131]. The school of Lamaze seems to take into account the teaching of the Kiev Congress. Thus, Vellay (1957) mentions the fundamental value of 'inhibition' or 'negative excitation'. Whereas Vermorel considers inhibitory activity as produced by analgesiant procedures, Vellay insists on the 'activity . . . obtained through rational education' which 'will *inhibit painful excitation*'.*

In his last work, in collaboration with Roelens, ANGELERGUES no longer insisted on the excitation–inhibition problem. He merely says about 'cortical activation', that woman must be taught 'every positive activity she will have to display at the various stages of delivery' [17].

There is also confusion with regard to the mode of action of neuromuscular education. This subject will be discussed when we compare the methods of Velvovski and Read later in chapter 11 (cf. p. 175).

As far as suggestion is concerned, the French theoreticians have almost exclusively followed Velvovski's view, categorically rejecting all suggestion. But since 1951 this standpoint has been frequently discussed in the USSR, and many different writers admit the importance of suggestion at all stages of the method. In 1956 at Kiev, these views were confirmed.

*Italics in the text.

French workers have underestimated the importance of the interpersonal relationship. Angelergues criticizes Read for producing a personal ascendancy over the women whom he prepared, 'this power essentially corresponds to certain phenomena of suggestion and hypnotism which only work below a certain level of consciousness'. LAMAZE also wrote in 1955, 'This preparation works only insofar as it is an education of the higher level of consciousness, very far removed from a series of suggestions, from some exercises or from a simple modification of the emotional environment. To really reassure the woman it is necessary to convince her and this necessitates in general explanations which are pushed much further than one would like to think' [296]. Lamaze also rejects suggestion and pronounces himself in favour of persuasion which, according to him, is the chief element in the preparation. This persuasion is even more important than the exercises and the emotional atmosphere.

This attitude of Lamaze recalls the position of the Swiss Psychotherapeutic School of Dubois (working in Berne) at the beginning of this century. DUBOIS was opposed to the idea of suggestion as it was put forward by Bernheim, and recommended a rational psychotherapy based on persuasion. He wrote in 1909: 'Many doctors wish, with all their might, to consider that the influence which I exercise on my patients springs from suggestion. Bernheim, in particular, has attempted in a series of publications, to defend his own work whilst confusing *suggestion* and *persuasion*.* These revindications of priority are unjustifiable because our methods are not only different but opposed' [136]. To this BERNHEIM [43] replied, 'Others pretend to have invented, in place of my suggestive psychotherapy, which they call thaumaturgic, a true psychological therapy which they consider the only rational one; then they do not call it suggestion any more but persuasion. . . .'

JANET also intervened in the controversy, and wrote 'Monsieur Dubois (of Berne) draws our attention to the fact that suggestion only addresses itself to the automatic tendencies of the patient and not to his reason, his will, to the *most elevated parts of his personality*,† and as it appears the automatic tendencies are lower than reason and will—here is a treatment which is, for him, therefore morally very much inferior' [247].

*Italics in the text. †Author's italics. (L.C.)

In 1957 Angelergues and Roelens recognized that suggestion produced successes in obstetrical analgesia, which proved the 'very great biological strength of speech'. But they consider that this strength is used at a 'relatively lower' level in suggestion. 'Why not direct it rationally', they say, 'at the level of the most complex educational processes, at the level of conscious phenomena, where speech plays precisely its most effective role?'

In reality it is difficult to dissociate the element of persuasion from that of suggestion, above all in medical practice. As regards analgesia, persuasion does not abolish nor diminish the pain. The diminution of obstetrical pain—if it is obtained by psychoprophylactic preparation—results from the psychological action (called suggestive psychotherapy or just psychotherapy) of the doctor on the pregnant woman. Psychological analgesia is an experimental fact, its physiological mechanism is still poorly understood, but it is certain that the pathway is emotional and unconscious, the equivalent to Janet's 'automatic tendency'. In consequence if there is an analgesia it is produced 'at a lower level' if by such a phrase the unconscious emotional life can be put into spatial relationship with the conscious. The physiotherapeutic and didactic elements are useful and necessary intermediaries, and a technique which is codified and systematized is indispensable. But preparation without an 'emotional relationship' is inoperative. An emotional relationship always exists in the phase of preparation, even if the person who is preparing the woman believes that it rests solely at the level of a 'persuasive' action.

Vermorel, taking count of the objections which have been voiced in the Soviet Union against Velvovski, believes that 'there exist elements of suggestion in the Psychoprophylactic Method, at the same time as there exist didactic elements', but he adds, 'it can be supposed that the first will go on diminishing and that the development of education more generally, and the extension of prophylaxis in particular, will allow us to remove, little by little, these elements of elementary suggestion, which will in time take only second place in the psychoprophylactic method'.

But why is there this discontent with suggestion? Suggestion, according to Pavlov, forms 'the most simple and the most typical of the conditioned reflexes of man'. Doubtless in the current usage of the term the word suggestion is often used in a depreciatory manner, but in a larger sense it can describe every psychological action of the doctor on his patient.

Later on, in 1957 ECONOMIDES and VERMOREL [143] defend themselves against the accusation that they misrepresent suggestion 'a scientific phenomenon of which the doctor ought to make use'. They add nevertheless, 'there are educational elements in the Psychoprophylactic Method and no one would consider that education was a sort of exaggerated suggestion'. They believe that the analgesiant mechanism in the educational factor is not clear and that 'one of the problems related to painless childbirth is that of consciousness'. In order to prove that suggestion is not predominant they mention the failure to use hypnosuggestive methods in general, and the great extension of the Psychoprophylactic Method.

It should be pointed out however that the inapplicability of the hypnosuggestive methods on a large scale is not due to their ineffectiveness. All authors agree in recognizing that on the contrary they are superior to the Psychoprophylactic Method and the Russian workers use them in particularly difficult cases. The inapplicability in question springs from different causes: the lack for instance of competent practitioners as well as the fact that it is a method which cannot be used by auxiliary personnel. Also conscious and unconscious resistances are aroused by any process involving the manipulation of emotion, and these resistances are shown just as much by the public as by doctors. Throughout its history hypnosis as any psychotherapy has been the object of passionate opposition and controversy.* In spite of certain elucidations that the teachings of Pavlov have produced at the physiological level, and by the Freudian theory at the psychological level, hypnosis still remains surrounded by a certain taboo.

*And this from the beginning, as it was seen as early as 1784 during the discussion in the Academies on 'Animal Magnetism'. This still occurs today. A meeting recently took place (February 1957) between Freudians and Pavlovians in Fribourg (Western Germany). The discussion, in which nearly 200 specialists took part, was fairly stormy, as can be judged from the report of Volgyesi, published in the *Korsakov Review of Neuro-Pathology and Psychiatry*. This author, a Hungarian hypnologist and author of the book *Die Seele ist alles* (The Soul is all) adopted an intransigent attitude, contrasting the followers of the psychologic, neuro-physiologic and materialistic psychiatric concep-

As for the relationship between education and suggestion, an identical mechanism does not seem to be present. It is clear that the analgesia operates by means of interpersonal relations (not only verbal ones). It is difficult to distinguish between a relationship of a suggestive nature and of an educational nature. The first is itself still very badly defined, the second brings in other elements. All that can be said for certain is that analgesia, produced by suggestion, is an experimental fact, whilst the analgesiant effect of 'rational understanding' remains uncertain.

This is not to say that education ought to be eliminated but only that it is always important to bear interpersonal relationships in mind, even if they are clothed in the form of elementary suggestion. In respect of this it is worth quoting AJURIAGUERRA'S [10] remarks made at the Symposium in Paris: 'Certain doctors deny that they use suggestion but in fact employ it without knowing it, making use of formulae whose magical character escapes them. It is always useful to cure or to relieve, even by suggestion. What appears to us antiscientific is to misunderstand the important value of the doctor/patient relationship and to obscure this in formulae which are often just as obscure. Even though one takes this attitude, suggestion is not therefore eliminated, and the understanding of the phenomenon is much diminished'.

To show the importance of the interpersonal relationship, even in the form of pure suggestion, it is enough to report the experiences of the pregnant women themselves. There are some very interesting passages in the book published by Dr. Vellay and Aline Vellay, *Témoignages sur l'Accouchement sans douleur*. Quotations such as this seem significant: 'The doctor encourages me by his voice, his look, and this co-operation between him and me is such that I had no longer the impression of being alone in pushing, and it was this which allowed me to produce the effort which was demanded of me' (p. 47). 'The doctor gave me his precise instructions, encouraging me by his words, imposing his will on me, directing me in the slightest details of the movements which I had to do. Moreover he (the doctor) helps you by his encouragement during labour so that you can push—and I still more than ever realize at this time the magic of rhythm and of the human voice which understands how to weld the rhythm

---

tions' with the western representatives of the 'millenary mystico-magic and idealistic-dualist approach'.

with the act that is to be accomplished' (p. 55). 'I could not see Mme D. any longer (the midwife). It seemed to me that she directed the whole universe; if she was away I felt ill; everything became peaceful in her presence—she is so pretty' (p. 73).

TSOULADZE and COENCA [541] consider that the two factors, education and suggestion, coexist in the method and that it is not important to choose between them but to use them in proportion, depending on the personality of the woman. This personality is considered in terms of Pavlov's Nervous Types and particularly with regard to the division in man into the artistic and the intellectual types. In the first, the first signalling system predominates—there is a lively emotionality, a thought charged with impulsive emotivity (symptomatology of hysterical type). In the second there is a tendency to reasoning, to mental operations by the use of words (in a pathological form this is the psychoasthenic type). There is an intermediate type between these two extreme types. With the artistic type suggestion has more effect whilst education has more effect in the intellectual type. Tsouladze and Coenca attempted to determine these types by means of tests used in Russia; the word association test modified by Gakkel and the suggestibility test of Hull or 'body sway test'. The pros and cons of these tests have already been remarked upon; the difficulties are recognized by the Russians quite clearly. But Tsouladze and Coenca introduce here a new idea when they point out that the results are influenced by *the Nervous Type of the doctor*. In fact they have been struck by the variability in the results obtained by the same technique used by different technicians.

To close this section devoted to theoretical developments in France, the interesting discussion which took place at the Symposium of 7 April 1957, will be briefly reported. This concerned the Pavlovian explanation of pain; in what respect can this explanation be extended to man?

NOTTER [404] has remarked that Pavlov's dogs, as Pavlov himself always stressed, were starved, and that the height of their hierarchy from the psychological point of view was represented by an appetizing meal. But it is somewhat different in the woman; speech, surely, cannot be considered as on the same level as a meal. This point was again taken up by AJURIAGUERRA [10], who stressed that in the animal there was an extremely long preparation for pain whilst human pain occurred by successive fits and starts and depended upon a general organization of the organism. He added, 'It is not only a functioning through an analyser in relationship to the cortex, it is a general organization of the cortex in relationship with an analyser. This is a vital fact.'

The discussion was then devoted to the second signalling system—speech. Ajuriaguerra criticized the tendency to make speech the be-all and end-all of psychology. For him there is something more general than speech and this is communication, which may just as well be non-verbal. It is also not sufficient to say that 'something happens in the second system' as an explanation; saying that, we are merely stating that the psychological factor exists, and this is precisely where the problem begins. Muldvorf remarked that the intersubjective relationship could not be substituted for language, and that it could not exist without language; Ajuriaguerra denied that he underestimated the verbal relationship. It is, he believes, essential but should be seen in the setting of a whole system of relations, of which the emotional relationship is just as important. A deaf and dumb mute could thus be delivered painlessly in the same way as a normal woman.

RESULTS

According to VERMOREL [561], the number of childbirths in France, in which the method was used, rose to more than 10,000 in 1955. At the Havana Conference in 1955, Lamaze presented the results which had been collected at the Polyclinique des Métallurgistes, bearing on 4847 childbirths. The results were as follows:

Excellent	893	18·43 per cent
Very Good	1097	22·63 ,, ,,
Good	1172	24·17 ,, ,,
Fair	859	17·73 ,, ,,
Poor	595	12·28 ,, ,,
Failures	231	4·76 ,, ,,

The French workers state they have obtained analogous results to those of the Russian workers, although it is difficult to assess this as the Russians use a four point scale. The results are based on the behaviour of the woman as observed by the obstetricians and the midwives, and on the woman's account as labour proceeds. 'They then take account,' writes Lamaze, 'of all the objective elements of the perception of uterine activities.' Nevertheless it is well known, and the Russian writers have often underlined this, that no objective criteria exist which allow us to measure pain sensation, and that the statements of the parturient woman are always subjective and of relative value. This does not prevent ANGELERGUES from writing 'Speech is an objective manifestation of the individual. ... All manifestations, whether motor or verbal, are objective, that is to say subject to a rigorous determinism, according to the laws of higher nervous activity. The individual expresses objectively, by words, the nervous process which is felt subjectively' [16]. But surely this is nothing but a mechanistic interpretation of speech and the writer is confusing the objective with the material.

ANGELERGUES also writes, believing in the 'objectivity' of the statements of the parturients,* that he has no hesitation in predicting 'the disappearance of pain' [18]. LAMAZE himself has declared [296] that 'the psychoprophylactic method is exactly aimed at abolishing pain, formerly said to be inevitable, which is bound up with the contraction of the uterus'. The Russian workers on the other hand have been careful to show no great optimism in this field, for this could bring the method into disrepute. For this reason they have considered it wiser not to stress the pain factor in their new nomenclature for the method. On a different level of analgesia LAMAZE and MULDVORF [306] studied 50 women by means of a lengthy questionnaire, after their childbirth. Their aim was to examine the psychological, psychotherapeutic and sociological aspects of painless childbirth. Seventy per cent of the women attached importance to the theoretical lessons. Twenty-four stated that they had got over the difficult periods of their labour 'not by the mechanical carrying out of the different adaptive activities but by rationally thinking over the whole of the preparation'.

The psychotherapeutic advantages are enormous and made themselves felt even in neuroses which had been present before the pregnancy. One of the women stated that she had benefited

*It is true that three years later, in 1957, Angelergues distinguished 'two orders of criteria, the ones called objective, the others called subjective' and specified that the latter are made up of the records of verbal evidence given by women about their feelings during delivery [18].

more by the psychoprophylactic preparation than by a long course of psychoanalytic treatment.

Lamaze and Muldvorf translated psychological terms into physiological language. For instance psychotherapy becomes 'a reorganization of the higher nervous activity through the medium of speech'. The will and knowing how to control it is nothing else than a matter of how best to improve the cortical processes.

As well as the publications coming from the Clinique des Métallurgistes, a great deal of work on the Psychoprophylactic Method has been carried out in France. In 1954, five dissertations were dedicated to this problem by DIETLIN (Bordeaux), THIS (Nancy), Coenca, Maurel and Roux (Paris.) In 1955 two by MALAGUTI [344] and SVARTZ [515] of Paris, and two in 1956 by DANTEC [111] and PRUDENT [440]. RIVIÈRE and CHASTRUSSE [468], of Bordeaux, have dealt with the problem of obstetrical psychoprophylaxis in their report on obstetrical pain given at the Second Congress of Gynaecologists and Obstetricians of the Mediterranean countries at Turin in May 1954.* In the same year COLETTE JEANSON published a popular book, *The Principles and Practice of Painless Childbirth* [250], and GAILLARD also published a brochure on *The Practice of Painless Childbirth* [184]. YMENET (1954) claims that the preparation for childbirth is the province of the physiotherapist. This necessitates, she says, a paramedical training, teaching capacity, and the ability to build up a good relationship with the patients, as well as a close cooperation with the obstetrician.

Results from the practice of the method have been published from 1954 on. RAVINA *et al.* (1954) carried out a theoretical review of the method and described the technique they used at the Maternity Hospital of Lariboisière. They analysed 30 cases, in 22 of whom successful results were obtained. LARRIBIÈRE (1954) in Oran studied 40 cases, whilst BAUX (1954) of Toulouse recorded his experiences in private practice. He had 60 good results. He considered that the panting respiration tired the women, dehydrating them and increasing their consumption of oxygen.

In 1955 he reported with Ferrier 700 cases in private practice [33]. The two writers insist on the incontestable superiority of

*Read's method was also dealt with in this report.

psychoprophylactic analgesia over the other methods of analgesia if one takes into account the good of the child. They believe that relaxation has an undoubted analgesiant effect. During the exercises numerous women go to sleep and then go through childbirth successfully without the least tendency to sleep during the delivery itself.*

Their results were as follows: 49·1 per cent complete success, 29·4 per cent partial success and 21·3 per cent failure.

They also studied the Nervous Types of the women but do not give their criteria for classification. Out of the 122 failures, 48 women were of the weak or unstable type whereas out of the 468 successful cases, only six were of this type.

ROLLAND and ROLLAND (1954) of the Hautes-Pyréneès, delivered 26 women in their homes in 1953, and 57 in 1954 using the psychoprophylactic method. FAVAREL (1955) of Rennes also studied the problem of the use of the psychoprophylactic method by the country doctor in the patient's home.

GOIRAND (1955) of Marseilles described one hundred cases and compared them with 100 controls who had had no preparation. Of the hundred who had not been prepared 73 suffered a good deal and of the women who had been prepared only 16 suffered. As for painless childbirths, he had five in the group who had no preparation and 39 in the group who had been prepared. He draws attention to the importance of the mental make-up of the doctor. A doctor who tries his hand at psychoprophylaxis, without believing in it, will have failures, because he will not be able to communicate the psychological feeling so necessary to the woman in childbirth.

CHAPUS [76] studied 30 women in his private practice and LE LORIER (1956) reported his experience of the method at the

---

*This is a very interesting observation. These women have passed through hypnoid states in the course of which, according to the Russian workers, suggestibility is increased. Baux and Ferrier seem to have no idea that it is on account of these hypnoid states that Velvovski has renounced relaxation, and considers that Read's method is one of hypnosis (cf. p. 179).

The absence of sleep during childbirth would not invalidate a post-hypnotic suggestive action (cf. Kogerer, p. 26). The personnel preparing the women doubtless do not give direct suggestions of analgesia during the exercises, but the exercises have a suggestive effect in themselves.

Clinique Baudelocque in Paris. He published a statistical analysis of the first hundred cases during a first trial period. Good results were obtained in 47 per cent, medium results in 36 per cent and 17 per cent were failures. He was only successful in obtaining 12 per cent of positive results with regard to analgesias.

VITTOZ-MEYNARD (1956) of Paris has studied 400 psychoprophylactic childbirths, of whom 300 received preparation. She obtained good results on 70 per cent, and also noted that in 84 multiparae who were not prepared, 45 per cent preserved a perfect, or nearly perfect, calm. During the course of the childbirth she made use of antispasmodics and oxytocics in small dosage. She considers that the lumbar* pains and the bone pains were often a cause of the failure of the method.

QUICHON (1957) of Besançon, has prepared 1000 women by the Psychoprophylactic Method. He also uses drugs such as spasmaverine and sparteine in moderate doses. He records that he had no need to use forceps and that the preparation exerted a favourable influence on lactation.

SCHEBAT (1956) of Algiers himself individually or collectively prepared 160 women (100 of whom were primiparae). He uses a combination of the Psychoprophylactic Method and induced labour. This consists of the early rupture of the membranes (when there is a two or three finger dilatation), and the injection of 250 mg of sparteine camphorate, either combined with 0·5 cm^3 of dolosal in primiparae or 0·5 cm^3 of spasmalgine in multiparae. He has had no cases where the child needed resuscitation.

GRANDALIANO-MOLLARD and ARLAUD (1956) of Marseilles have delivered 1000 women in a private hospital by the psychoprophylactic method.

*The problem of lumbar pain is important. Le Lorier believes that these pains form the chief stumbling block of the psychoprophylactic method, for it is practically powerless against them. Lumbar massage also hardly helps them at all. Of a 100 cases he studied, he found these pains in about a third of his cases [318].

BURTHIAULT and GARNIER [69] of Lyon also maintain that lumbar pains are important causes of failure. They consider that they occur throughout the pregnancy, and have a mechanical cause; they can be alleviated by physiotherapy. WERRA and DUBUIS [574] found lumbar pain in 46 per cent of their cases, the majority coming on during childbirth.

GAVEL (1956) of Angoulême has made a study of psycho-prophylactic childbirth in small centres. He has dealt with 48 cases, and believes 'that psychoprophylactic childbirth is a technique which morally one has no longer the right to refuse, provided that the indications have been correctly assessed, just as with any other medical technique'.

COTTEEL et al. (1956) of Lille have carried out 268 deliveries in private practice using the psychoprophylactic method over a period of 18 months. They mention one important point: certain women refuse anaesthesia because they want to see their child born. They report that on one occasion foetal death resulted from a prolonged labour, when the mother refused a needed anaesthetic. It is therefore important to prepare the women for the eventuality of narco-anaesthesia.*

ROUCHY (1957) of Angers uses psychoprophylaxis in association with a wide range of drugs. ZAIDMAN (1957) reports on 182 cases which he has prepared since 1955 in the Municipal Health Centres of Argenteuil, Blanc-Mesnil and Nanterre. The deliveries took place in different maternity clinics in Paris. ECONOMIDES and VERMOREL (1957) report their experience with 380 cases.

In many other papers than those we have mentioned numerous theoretical points and clinical facts are dealt with.† (1954: LACOMME [290], LE LORIER [317], GRASSET and DUMONT [200], LANTUEJOUL and MERGER [289], LAMBERT [287]. In 1955: VERMELIN [522], LANTUEJOUL [310], GAILLARD [184], SIMON [506], LECOMTE [315], DECHAUME [116], GRASSET and DUMONT [199]. In 1956: ECONOMIDES [142], CHERTOK [82].)

RESULTS IN COUNTRIES OUTSIDE FRANCE

In Belgium, GREGOIRE (1956) also comes out in favour of painless childbirth. He believes that pain can be one of the causes of functional dystocia and can prolong delivery and even produce postnatal psychological complications for the woman. As with many other writers he draws attention to the danger of anaesthetics and analgesics both for the mother and for the child.

The Psychoprophylactic Method which has been 'adapted to

*Levy, of Paris also insists on this point.

†Some writers limit themselves to the study of the psychoprophylactic method, others also consider the English method.

occidental psychology by Dr. Lamaze', appeared to him more scientific because it draws on facts from experimental physiology.

At the psychological level, he recognizes masochistic tendencies in women and believes that it is necessary to 'divert these tendencies on to the efforts which should be made to learn how delivery should take place'.

DRAPS and SCHOYSMAN (1957), two Belgian practitioners, used the Psychoprophylactic Method in one thousand deliveries. PEETERS (1958) of Turnhout, made some interesting observations in his study on the use of R.875, a new analgesic, in obstetrics. First, he noted that the activity of R.875 largely depends on the surroundings and the nervous condition of the parturient woman. Nervous people were thus unaffected by the activity of R.875. Women prepared by the Psychoprophylactic Method who behaved calmly were not given R.875, but it was given to the non-prepared and to prepared women showing little result. The best results occurred amongst the latter group, who received R.875 as a complement to the preparation. For non-prepared women he advises a kind of extemporaneous psychoprophylactic preparation: a restful environment, explanations about labour, short periods of learning respiratory exercises, and constant presence during the critical period of labour.

It is still too early to give a definite opinion on the analgesic action and the possible side effects of R.875. We think it useful to stress two aspects of Peeters' work: the usefulness of R.875 as a complement to preparation; the importance of the psychological factor even when analgesic drugs are used.

In the Netherlands, DE LEEUWE (1955) is a fervent partisan of the method. In Switzerland, DE WATTEVILLE of Geneva [571–573], is an enthusiast for psychoprophylaxis. He was at first interested in Read's method. But he has found his results have been less satisfying, and considers that the woman remains too passive, and does not collaborate in her childbirth. Following a visit by Lamaze, he was struck by the logic and by the soundness of the theoretical basis of this system, where relaxation is of less importance than conditioning. His co-worker, GEISENDORF [188], after a visit to the Clinique des Métallurgistes in Paris, took the initiative in organizing psychoprophylactic preparation at the maternity unit in Geneva. In March 1955 the number of women who had been delivered had grown to a hundred. Twenty-five per cent had felt no pain, 50 per cent felt some slight pain; in 25 per cent the results were less satisfying.

In November 1956, DE WATTEVILLE [572] reported on 700 cases with similar results. He points out that there is a difference in the interpretation of the results as between the doctor and the nursing staff. The latter are more optimistic in the period of dilatation when the woman, whilst remaining calm, might feel disagreeable sensations. During the delivery the nursing personnel often notice groans and signs of agitation, even though afterwards the woman maintains that she has not suffered at this particular time. DE WATTEVILLE maintains that the psychoprophylactic preparation 'has allowed about three-quarters of the women to go through the phase of dilatation easily, without analgesia, and almost nine-tenths of them are able to have a painless period without anaesthesia during the second stage of parturition'. He believes that there has been an almost revolutionary diminution in the administration of nitrous oxide and that the use of chloroform can almost be abandoned. On the other hand he did not notice any reduction in the length of labour nor in the number of obstetrical interventions that were made.

Comparing anew Read's method with the psychoprophylactic method, at the Conference of the American Society of Obstetricians and Gynaecologists in 1956, DE WATTEVILLE stated that there is no fundamental difference between the two methods [573]. He nevertheless still believes that Read's method appeals to the woman's passivity, whilst the Psychoprophylactic Method appeals to the patient's activity.

ROUX and DE WATTEVILLE (1957) have studied the intelligence level of women undergoing the Psychoprophylactic Method. They state that women of higher intelligence level have a greater chance of success. They are therefore inclined to believe 'that the faculty of acquiring conditioned reflexes depends on the intellectual level'.

GEISENDORF (1957), a fervent partisan of the Psychoprophylactic Methods, pays particular attention to the psychosomatic aspects. He says 'it is heartrending to see the psychosomatic behaviour of a certain number of *accoucheurs* who have still not understood the interest of the method, its social value and its physical advantages, both for the mother and the newborn child'. He stresses that doctors ought, amongst themselves, to be convinced and enthusiastic; otherwise the method is likely to fail. As to those who do not take part personally in the preparation 'they deprive themselves of a great joy and of a precious contact with the patients whom they will eventually deliver'.

GEISENDORF not only recommends a psychological contact between the doctor and the patient, but he also believes that this contact can be reinforced by an active participation—a 'somatic' participation of the doctor. He recommends for this a technique which he claims to have practised regularly with primaparae for more than 20 years. It consists essentially for the doctor, standing to the right of the bed, 'to offer his left hip to the woman so that she can put her right foot on it and to take her right hand in his right hand'. The midwife plays a similar part on the other side of the bed.*

NORDMANN [400] at Fribourg also used the Psychoprophylactic Method and by 1955 had had experience in a hundred cases. In Lausanne, ROCHAT (1955) is an enthusiastic partisan of the method, which he considers different from that of Read. Of the Psychoprophylactic Method he writes that 'it is not just another method which is added to other analgesic procedures which are already known. It is not too much to say that it is a complete change in the history of childbirth'. He very much insists on the active role, on the positive and conscious attitude of the woman which 'directs' her childbirth. It seems, however, that he only partly agrees with Velvovski. For ROCHAT the aim of the respiratory exercises is the oxygenation of the uterine muscle, in contradistinction to the views of Russian writers, who maintain that they chiefly serve as procedures which reduce cortical pain through the mechanism of attention. Rochat has studied 110 cases, 25 per cent with excellent results, 25 per cent with very good and 25 per cent with good results. He had 10 per cent of failures and in 15 per cent there was a moderate result.

With Rossel he reports almost similar results on 400 cases between 1 May 1955 and 30 April 1956 [436]. These 400 cases 248 primiparae, 152 multiparae) were drawn from a total of 1553

---

*DAVIDSON [113] reports a similar procedure practised and taught in the beginning of the century by Professors Voorhees and Caldwell of Columbia University.

deliveries carried out at the University Maternity Clinic of Lausanne. The authors stress in particular the importance of painless childbirth for the foetus: 3·25 per cent of resuscitations were found in the women who had been prepared as against nine per cent in those who had not been prepared. It should be noted that in Switzerland the importance of painless childbirth has been officially recognized, as shown by a decree of the Grand Council ordering the creation of a division for painless childbirth at the Maternity Clinic of the University of Lausanne.

Two other Swiss writers, DE WERRA and DUBUIS (1956) in one year delivered 164 women in their private practice. They themselves prepared the women. They stress the almost total disappearance of resuscitations needed for the baby (only a slight resuscitation was needed in two cases). Forceps application without anaesthesia was practised with success in four cases because the woman 'would feel frustrated of the essential part of the adventure, just as might the mountain climber who, at the very moment when, after enormous physical effort, he has attained a most remarkable viewpoint, would there and then bandage his eyes'. The psychological results are difficult to assess. The essential to these authors in this respect is 'the change in the total climate of the pregnancy, in the whole atmosphere surrounding the childbirth, and the total transformation of the attitude of the woman towards her delivery. These women are relaxed, docile, happy and this alone would be enough to justify the use of this method'.

BERLOZ (1956), reports on his experience of the psychoprophylactic method in a small hospital in the district of La Vallée. With two midwives he delivered 41 women in the second half of 1955.

MEYLAN [365], believes that Read's method is based on passivity, and the Psychoprophylactic Method on activity.

After spending some time at the Polyclinique des Métallurgistes in Paris in 1953, the psychiatrist SEABRA-DINIS [502, 503], became a fervent adherent of the Psychoprophylactic Method in Portugal. He collaborated with the obstetricians MONJARDINO [372] and VICENTE [562] at the Hospital de l'Ultramar at Lisbon. In May 1956 586 women had undergone psychoprophylactic preparation in this unit. In Portugal studies have also been published on the method by BERMUDES [41], and DOS SANTOS [134]. MEDEIROS

[360], in her thesis, describes her own psychoprophylactic childbirth. Cota Guerra has been using the method in Mozambique. BARAHONA FERNANDEZ [31] of Lisbon has several reservations of a theoretical nature concerning the reflexological explanations of the method.

In Spain HERNANDEZ JIMENEZ (1957), after visiting the Clinique des Métallurgistes in 1953, has carried out the Psychoprophylactic Method in his practice at the Santa Alicia clinic in Madrid. In 1957 he reported his results, only, however, in percentages. He had excellent results in 32 per cent, good in 21 per cent, fair in 28 per cent, failures 19 per cent. He mentions a peculiarity of the local customs which makes psychoprophylactic childbirth a delicate problem. In Spain the whole family assists and comforts the parturient woman during the phase of dilatation. For this reason training ought to be extended to the whole family. As to the collaboration of the husband, he believes that this is absolutely desirable. He goes so far as to say that the successful cases have been obtained largely thanks to the collaboration of the husband; when this was missing the method has failed either completely or partially. But this collaboration being difficult to obtain in practice, Hernandez-Jimenez sees in this the reason for the relatively high number of failures. He mentions, moreover, that the Psychoprophylactic Method is applied by other Spanish practitioners: by ORENGO and LUQUE in Madrid; PUIG ROIG, CORNILL, RODES and DEXEUS in Barcelona; DERQUI in Valencia; UCIEDA in Leon and many others.

Since 1954, MALCOVATI [345] has carried out the Psychoprophylactic Method as taught at the Clinique des Métallurgistes, together with his collaborators CORNALI, MIRAGLIA, ORLANDINI, Micheletti and others. He works at the Provincial Institute of Maternity in Milan, the most important in Italy (having an average of 13 births a day). He is the director of this hospital but works as well in other hospitals in the town. His figures relate to 2000 cases, in 40 per cent of whom the results were excellent, 30 per cent very good, 10 per cnet good, 8 per cent fair, and 12 per cent were failures. He claims that there is a reduction in the mean length of labour, of the number of obstetrical interventions which are necessary, as well as in a diminution in the number of foetal disturbances. His team are carrying out oxymetric investigations during childbirth. Using Thorn's tests they have demonstrated that childbirth has a more stressing action in women who have not been prepared than amongst those who have been prepared. Electroencephalographic studies have been made during the preparation but they present difficulties in technique which have so far been insurmountable. Psychological tests have been made also in collaboration with the doctors at the Institute of Psychology of the Catholic University of Milan.

Other cities such as Rome, Bologna, Naples and Genoa have followed the example of Turin and Milan in introducing psychosomatic methods of painless childbirth. The Psychoprophylactic Method has also spread in South America.

CHAPTER 11

A COMPARISON OF THE METHODS OF READ AND VELVOVSKI

A PASSIONATE controversy has taken place concerning the relationship between the methods of Read and Velvovski; some deny that there is any relationship, others maintain that one is similar to the other. In 1953, LAMAZE and VELLAY [298] inveighed against those who differentiated between the two methods 'as if there could exist two different methods of painless childbirth produced by psychophysical methods'. They also criticized those who held that Read's discoveries preceded those in Soviet Russia. 'These are miserable arguments, tainted with the most mediocre partisan spirit!' Pavlov, they recalled, was frequently quoted by Read. They recognized that 'the results Read obtained cannot be disputed', they are analogous to those of Soviet workers. They recalled that the Americans, notably Thoms at Yale, and the Canadians, using Read's technique, had themselves produced painless childbirth by psychophysical means. But about 1954 their views changed. Lamaze, for example, wrote 'It seems essential for us to define in what way the Pavlovian method of painless childbirth produced by psychoprophylaxis differs completely from other known psychological methods, known or disseminated under the names of "Childbirth without Fear" (Read), "Natural Childbirth", etc.' [301]. Vermorel even considers that there ought to be no question of comparing 'two methods which are not even on the same level, one empirical and the other scientific'.

Before describing the French criticisms of Read, it is well to mention an error frequently found in regard to his work, that it began after the inauguration of the Russian method. Thus ANGELERGUES writes 'Read began his work on the suppression of the pain of childbirth ten years later than Russian doctors' [16]. In fact, Velvovski's first publications on psychoprophylaxis appeared in 1949, whilst Read's first book was published in 1933. Angelergues picked out 1923 as the beginning of the Russian work, but in fact this was the time when hypnosuggestive methods were being used in Russia, not the Psychoprophylactic Method. Indeed, on this count, the Russian work had been preceded, 60 years or more previously, by the experiments of LAFONTAINE [291] and LIÉBAULT [329] on the use of hypnosis in obstetrical analgesia. Vermorel, however, recognized that Read's method antedated that of Velvovski, but considered that it represented 'a stage in the history of obstetrical analgesia following hypnosis and before psychoprophylaxis'.*

The criticisms of French writers bear on the following points.

1. *The empiricism of the method.* It is true that Read's conception

---

*LACOMME [290] has given an historical account of the practice of these psychosomatic methods in France.

'The technique was developed and laid down by an English accoucheur, Dick Read, whose first publications date from 1929. I have searched in vain for a reference to it in the French literature. It seems that, in general, Read met with little credence, and his idea only slowly made its mark. However, just before the war, Lévy-Solal, at St. Antoine became interested and even made a film on natural childbirth. In spite of its well-known author, this attempt met with little response.

'In 1947, Dick Read, three years after the publication of his second book, entitled more modestly than his first *Childbirth without Fear*, no longer *Natural Childbirth*, himself gave a lecture at the Clinique Tarnier, on the invitation of Professor Lantuéjoul; its reception was still lukewarm. Not that the method was thought to be without interest, but it must be said that the majority of French obstetricians either read or listened to Read very sceptically. "One can't believe in it, or hardly at all", it was said. Some thought that in the relationship between the doctor and his patient during pregnancy, "confidence was slowly built up, thus producing a very useful psychotherapy". We all know how just coming into the room of a woman in labour will help to produce calm in the patient. Fear certainly produces, in many women, more crying than pain itself. The presence of the obstetrician she needs does not ease her suffering, but it disperses her anxiety and brings her an undeniable relief.

'Our experience, at the lecture of the English obstetrician, suggested that for long we had been doing what Read had done, without knowing it. And, in fact, many of us did not think it was possible to obtain much more by applying his complete technique. We were probably wrong. Probably we failed to apply the method with enough conviction, and in a large enough series. The systematic and convincing application has come from Russia, and their results, described with insistence and energy, and accompanied by explanatory physiological theory has overcome our scepticism.'

of the triad fear–tension–pain is debatable from the physiological point of view. Nevertheless, the physiological basis of the Psychoprophylactic Method is still far from being definitely established. Read and Velvovski agree on the same postulate—the painless character of natural childbirth, which ethnological study has not confirmed. But Velvovski has the merit of having taken into consideration an experimentally valid fact, analgesia produced by hypnotic suggestion.

2. *His conception of relaxation.** French workers believe that the neuromuscular release which they practise has a different aim from that of Read. Read's method leads to a state of inhibition, to a lowering of consciousness (whilst, following Read, his method ought to allow the woman to take an active part in childbirth). Practically, as the exercises are similar in both methods, it is relevant to ask in what way their modes of action can be different. The problem is confused. For the Russians relaxation is based on inhibition, and as such excluded in the usual preparation, and reserved for difficult cases which need particular attention. In the French psychoprophylactic technique relaxation is still included, and Angelergues recognizes that 'the state of muscular release corresponds, from the neurological point of view, to a state of inhibition'. But, in the Psychoprophylactic Method, the inhibition is not enough, muscular release is used to obtain an excitatory reinforcement, through a central activation.

BOURREL et al. [58] consider that the muscular release is an active phenomenon. They warn the women that they will not be trained in a state of rest, of somnolence, and still less of sleep. On the other hand BAUX and FERRIER's studies [33] (cf. p. 166), as we have set it out, have put forward evidence for the existence of hypnoid states. Such states are seen in the women who go to sleep during the exercises and then go through labour in excellent condition.

On the other hand it is perfectly true that Read himself, at the start, spoke of a passive state of relaxation which should be adopted throughout the contractions, but his followers (Heardman, Goodrich) emphasize the action factor. Goodrich even considers that during the phase of advanced dilatation it is necessary to use relaxation cautiously because it is accompanied

*The problem of relaxation will be discussed in Chapter 12.

by a tiring activity.* Read himself speaks of a concentration 'on the relaxation' [464].

3. *His results.* French writers consider that in this regard there is an essential difference, because Read's method is one of childbirth without fear, and Velvovski's one of childbirth without pain. Vermorel believes that the goal of Read's followers in France is not a complete analgesia, which is considered to be Utopian, but a diminution of the pain. He even accuses them of producing 'a true counter-psychoprophylaxis', because they deny the reality of painless childbirth, and consider that it would be dangerous and wrong to follow those who claim complete success (MAYER and BONHOMME [357]).

Vermorel also criticizes Langevin-Droguet for writing 'Painless childbirth is an inexact expression because this method of psychophysical preparation does not completely suppress the pains. It diminishes them appreciably in certain cases; in others it helps to support them better; in yet others, it only brings a minimal, or even no, relief'.

The objections are no longer tenable after the Kiev Congress, at which the Russians, with five years' experience, declared that complete analgesia ought not to be claimed, or the method would be in danger of being discredited.

The attempts to differentiate between the two methods have not convinced other French practitioners. For the most part they consider the difference is minimal. In 1954 LACOMME [290], for example, writes 'The main lines of the technique already laid down by Read do not seem to have been appreciably modified by the Russian doctors and obstetricians, Platonov, Velvovski, Plotitcher and Chougom who have more recently listed them.' RIVIÈRE and CHASTRUSSE [468] also consider 'One cannot escape the striking similarity between the Read method and that of the Russians. This is found both in the preparation, educational, psychological and physical, and in the conduct of labour itself. The slight differences in detail cannot destroy the impression of an almost perfect correspondence between the two methods.'

LYONNET [341] sees a difference in the methods, believing that 'education is more physical than mental in Read's technique' and

*It could be said that the relaxation during the contractions is a 'pain-reducing procedure', as understood by the Russians.

that 'on the other hand it is principally mental in the Russian method'. 'In fact I believe,' he says, 'that it is more in keeping with the character of the majority of French women to appeal to the mind rather than to the musculature'.

At the Symposium on 7 April 1957, LAMAZE and VELLAY [305] also held that 'Read's method is only one stage in the development of the psychoprophylactic method'. They maintained that there should be no confusion between the two methods, and it seemed to them that it was deceitful to practise a different method under cover of the psychoprophylaxis of painless childbirth.

In Switzerland, some workers (de Watteville, Rochat) consider that the methods are different, whilst others (Merz) consider them the same. The Dutchman VAN EPS [148] practises Read's method, but the title of his paper brings in the word 'psychoprophylaxis'. After visiting the Clinique des Métallurgistes in Paris, and studying the practice of the Psychoprophylactic Method, he considers that it is identical to that of Grantly Dick Read. As has been noted previously (p. 70) these two methods tend to become more and more linked in practice. Thus, the practitioners of the Psychoprophylactic Method at the Clinique des Métallurgistes in Paris use relaxation, one of the chief elements in Read's method, although they interpret the mode of its action quite differently. Moreover, the respiratory exercises used by Lamaze and his followers are also used by certain practitioners of Read's method.

The Russian workers have hardly taken part in this debate. It was only in 1957 that they began to do so. In a communication sent to the Symposium on 7 April 1957 in Paris, Velvovski maintained that Read's method was essentially a hypnosuggestive method, owing to the use of relaxation, and the passivity which that implies.* 'What Read calls relaxation is nothing else than a typical hypnotic state'. This form of relaxation has been carried out in 1920–30–41 in Russia during 'the hypnosuggestive period, with the difference that this technique was based on the materialistic teaching of Pavlov'.

He then recalls that the essential factor in the Psychoprophylactic Method is the educational one.† He also points out other

*Relaxation is not always passive.
†Read himself has recently stressed that education is the most important factor in his method.

theoretical differences which separate it from the method of Read. 'Fears and negative emotions are not for us the unique and determining cause of the pain. . . . We believe they rest on the foundation of neurodynamic situations; they considerably increase unfavourable neurodynamic situations and complicate them'.*

But Velvoski shares with Read the fundamental idea that 'the pain of childbirth is neither eternal nor necessary for the normal conduct of this natural act; moreover it can be prevented'. At the same time the Russian worker warmly congratulates Dr. Read, whom he greets as 'a humanist of great spirit and noble heart'. Rather than stressing the points which separate us Velvovski writes, 'it is preferable to insist on all that binds us together in this great mission which consists in the liberation of millions and millions of women from suffering'. Velvovski does not, however, admit any similarity between the two techniques, but it is apparent that his point of view is not shared by a large number of Soviet obstetricians, at least amongst the better known. A striking example of this can be seen in the recent article which has appeared in No. 2, 1957, of the review *Obstetrics and Gynaecology* published by the Ministry of Public Health of the Soviet Union. The article, which deals with Natural Childbirth, is the work of an Australian, Dr. A. H. DOBBIN, of Melbourne [128].

He describes his technique, which was inspired by the work of Read, who, according to him, had 'begun, since 1931, to use in his obstetrical practice in England a method impregnated with Pavlov's ideas'. Dobbin's technique does not differ essentially from the usual educational methods encompassing didactic, physiotherapeutic, and psychotherapeutic elements. He insists on the active participation of the husband who takes part in certain sessions in the preparation. At some maternity units in Melbourne the husband is present during the first phase of childbirth and in some even at the birth itself. He recommends that the child should be put to the breast several minutes after the birth. This procedure produces a uterine contraction, a reduction of postnatal haemorrhage and the speeding up of the separation and expulsion of the placenta. The day following the birth the mother is allowed to get up. The child stays in its cot all day next to its

*'The neurodynamic situations' of Velvovski are discussed on p. 103.

mother, and for the first five days the husband and the mother are alone allowed to visit. From the sixth day onwards any visitor is allowed and on the eighth or ninth day the woman goes home.

In conclusion Dobbin writes, 'A rapid study of the theory and practice of the Psychoprophylactic Method as it is used in the Soviet Union has not convinced me of any essential difference between this method and the method of Natural Childbirth as it is practised in Australia'.

Following this article the Editorial Board of the Review published a statement which reads as follows, 'Dobbin's article is of great interest. Nevertheless it is not possible to subscribe to certain of his views, such as his idea that the husband should be allowed to be present during the childbirth, the immediate nursing of the child, the premature getting up of the mother, the visits of her parents and friends to the hospital'. The similarity between the techniques of Read and of psychoprophylaxis put forward by Dobbin was not contested by the editorial staff of the Review (which consist of very distinguished Soviet obstetricians such as Belochapko, Stepanov, Syrovatko and Figournov). If this were so the end would be in sight of the sterile battle which has been waged between the adherents of the Psychoprophylactic Method and that of Read. Then only would it be possible to direct every scrap of energy toward a solution of the problem. However, we should not be too optimistic. In the review, *Obstetrics and Gynaecology* No. 4, 1957, Syrovatko published an article in which the two methods are again opposed. He writes 'Read's method is essentially a hypnosuggestive method: the woman is in a state of relaxation, amnesia and exaltation. The Soviet method is based on an elevated psychomatic tone of the woman and on her active and conscious participation. In this way the Soviet method of psychoprophylactic, preparation is basically different from Read's method' (Table 2).

In the next issue, NICOLAIEV [392] also criticized Read's method by taking up the arguments of Lamaze's School, with special reference to those given by ANGELERGUES [15, 16]. In Nicolaiev's opinion Read rightly admitted that environmental influences might create negative conditioned reflexes in the pregnant woman. He also emphasized the importance of fear and the necessity of preparing women for childbirth. But in Read's technique, continues Nicolaiev, analgesia is accompanied by a lowering in the level of consciousness. Read failed to understand the preponderant role of the cortex, the conditioned reflex mechanisms, the roles of the second signalling system of signalization and the possibility of the modification of conditioned reflexes by preparation (this modification being an active process). Read believes that pain is formed in the thalamus. He had remained dualistic and mystic, but Nicolaiev salutes him as a courageous pioneer of eeinless childbirth.

Angelergues for his part, in a study published in 1957 with Roelens, does not recognize the similarity of the techniques, but adopts a slightly more moderate attitude. Read had, he thought, like the French followers of Charcot and Bernheim 'fought the dogma of the inevitability of pain in childbirth and had elaborated a method enabling him to obtain a very significant decrease of pain in childbirth. Sometimes he attains its nearly complete suppression, by some physiological procedures, inducing neurodynamic changes, and by a psychotherapy strongly impregnated with mysticism.'*

Angelergues considered that if the hypnotic methods and Read's method could not be used more widely, it was because they were lacking a 'rational conception of pain related to uterine contraction'. They 'underwent an ideological deterioration and fell to the level of magical practices'. It should be noted here that in the Soviet Union the hypnosuggestive method, far from degenerating into a magical practice, has encouraged many investigations inspired by Pavlov's theories, has given birth to the Psychoprophylactic Method, and is itself still practised today.

Angelergues believes that if Read's method has attained a new popularity in France during recent years since the introduction of the Psychoprophylactic Method, it is due to the 'rational core of the latter method which progressively, although incompletely, penetrated it'. Whatever the present differences between the methods, Angelergues states that 'there is a scientific movement which will necessarily lead to the unity of obstetrical analgesia'.

*In another study, ANGELERGUES [16] admits that 'it is possible to create powerful centres of cortical activity by purely mystical themes. It should be remarked that, physiologically speaking, the focus of excitation, when it is "analgesiant" is indifferent to the theme which created it, whether mystical or not. . . .'

Table 2. The Different Techniques Compared

Technique of	Information	Psychotherapy (suppression of fear and a good relationship)	Physical exercises	Respiration	During preparation	Relaxation Between contractions	During contractions
Read	+	+	+	+(2)	+(5)	—(8)	+(11)
Velvovski	+	+	—(1)	+(3)	—(6)	—(9)	—
Lamaze	+	+	—	+(4)	+(7)	±(10)	+(12)

(1) Physical exercises have been recommended by Nicolaiev since 1956.

(2) Deep respiration during the pregnancy leading to good oxygenation. Rapid respiration 25 per minute during contractions, at the phase of advanced dilatation. This form of breathing is first mentioned in 1955 in *Antenatal Illustrated* [464]. Panting respiration during the delivery itself.

(3) Deep rhythmical respiration during contractions—'pain reducing procedure=diversion of attention=cortical activation. Other procedures of the same nature: abdominal effleurage and deep pressure.

(4) Deep respiration as in the Velvovski technique. Shallow and fast respiration from the beginning of advanced dilatation (procedure introduced by Lamaze). Explanations given: oxygenation and cortical activation.

(5) Progressive relaxation (Jacobson's technique) although its use is not recognized as correct by the latter. 'Physical and mental' relaxation, concentration on relaxation, one can also fall asleep.

(6) Relaxation with a central action in the form of 'relaxing rest', propitious state (hypnoid) toward the strengthening of pain reducing procedures' by reiterated repetition (increased suggestibility). This exercise first practised in all the women under preparation is now reserved for difficult cases.

(7) The technique similar to that of Read.

(8) Mental relaxation=rest.

(9) Plotitcher recommended in 1954: local muscular release—closing of the eyes to avoid the loss of energy.

(10) Optional up to three-finger dilatation, useful afterwards.

(11) Active relaxation (physical, conscious) implying a concentration and controlled respiration.

(12) Active relaxation combined with respiratory exercises.

CHAPTER 12

AN EXAMINATION OF THE PROBLEMS

In the course of the preceding chapters, the history, the practice and the theory of the different methods of psychologically produced analgesia has been described. At this stage a more systematic review may be rewarding. We shall consider successively a number of problems, although this approach is somewhat artificial, as some of those problems are closely linked one with another. But it is used here for convenience.

1. PAIN

'For psychophysiology, pain, in its extreme complexity, appears as one of the most difficult of problems, the most studied and the most discussed'. Thus PIERON [416] began his paper at the Congress of Psychology in Stockholm in 1951, a survey of the results of researches into the psychophysiology of pain. Leriche in his last book, *Bases de la Chirurgie Physiologique*, has written, 'I have tried for many years to define a pathological anatomy of pain. It is a chimera which I have had to give up; there is no precise anatomical state underlying pain'. In inaugurating the symposium on pain at the Salpêtrière in 1955, the famous surgeon also said, 'What is pain? alas, we do not know. If we only knew exactly what it was, we would have less hesitations and fewer failures in our therapies'. He continued, 'What is the lesion, what is the functional state which underlies the sensation of cutting, pinching, biting or tearing? I do not know, but this diversity of expression leads me to think that pain is not a ready-made entity which is mediated by the pathways conducting sensibility'. He concluded by saying that pain 'can still be considered as a subject for research, and that the real therapy of pain will come one day from the knowledge which will have been acquired of what is today nothing but a group of unknown facts'.

It is difficult to define pain, and Ajuriaguerra in his masterly report concerning the integration of pain at the Symposium on 7 April 1957, chose the definition put forward by ROF CARBALLO [473]: 'Pain, as well as being a perception, is a reaction, and at the same time an expression (particularly individualized, and different from one subject to another) and an emotional manifestation which depends on the previous experiences in the history of the subject. The centrifugal reactions which accompany it are integrally linked with the pain'.

It is not intended to give a detailed survey of the psycho-physiological facts concerning pain. The pathways for the conduction of pain, well-known up to the thalamus, become more obscure in the thalamo-cortical regions, and it would not be useful to discuss them here. The most difficult problem, the most controversial and the most obscure, concerns the central representation of pain. PIERON [416], for example, considers that the essential role is played by the thalamus, whilst the Pavlovians believe that cortical activity is dominant. Recent discoveries concerning the physiological role of the brain stem reticular formation have opened new vistas in our understanding of this central mechanism.

The problem of the central production of pain is complicated enough when peripheral stimulation is involved, but much more complicated when pain occurs in the absence of peripheral stimulation, such as in psychological pains, psychalgias, and causalgias, of which so little is known. Masochism provides another problem, for here there is a perversion of pain perception: peripheral excitation normally followed by pain is transformed into a feeling of pleasure. The relationship between affectivity and pain is obvious. For example, together with ABOULKER and CAHEN we have made a study of women suffering from pains in the uro-genital region [83]. These were found to have a symbolic value; it was difficult to deny their relationship with emotional complexes. The elucidation of the psychosomatic problem of pain is one aspect of the whole problem of consciousness. This leads to a consideration of the relationship between physiology and psychology, a central problem, not only for modern medicine, but for all psychological and philosophical researches. Pavlov, for instance, wrote 'I am convinced that an important stage in human thought is approaching, when the physiological and the psychological, the objective and the subjective, will actually be fused'. Freud was also preoccupied with this problem for many years. In 1895 he wrote *The Essentials of a Scientific Psychology*, then abandoned his attempts. Later he several times returned to the question of the connections between psychological and physical processes, without being able to resolve them, but each time indicating that a psychoanalytic terminology would be, one day, replaced by a physiological terminology.

The complexity of the problem has been highlighted recently in the course of two international meetings; in 1953 [516] at the International Symposium on Brain Mechanisms and Consciousness at Montreal, and in 1955 [98] at the international conference at Marseilles on the electrical activity of the brain in relation to psychological phenomena. Physiologists and psychologists together have not been able as yet to breach the gap which exists between their two respective disciplines. The recent discoveries concerning the reticular formation have not as yet produced a resolution of the problem of the anatomico-physiological substratum of consciousness. The hypothesis of the connection of consciousness with the activities of the brain stem was not accepted by all the participants in the meeting at Montreal. GOURVITCH [196], a Russian author, describing this conference, considered that it was very stimulating, of great interest and would lead to further studies. 'The idea,' he writes, 'of an action exerted by subcortical centres on the cerebral cortex, is nothing new for Soviet workers, the numerous experimental facts reported at the conference only confirm the truth of Pavlov's hypothesis'. 'But theoretical considerations', continues Gourvitch, 'in particular the attempts to link up consciousness with the activity of the brain stem, were not convincing.' He regrets that 'the rich material which has come from Pavlov's laboratories, and those of his school dealing directly with this question were completely ignored during the discussion on the relationships between consciousness and cerebral structure'. It is interesting, too, to relate the opinion of HUGELIN [238], a pupil of Dell, who adopts a cautious attitude. 'It is not for the physiologist to define consciousness, but he can perhaps say that consciousness requires two mechanisms; one a cortical analyser, the other a reticular dynamism, and that the activity of the second is a condition *sine qua non* of the activity of the first'. As to Magoun, the discoverer of the activity of the reticular formation, he recognized that the 'Symposium on brain mechanisms and consciousness' was a step forward, but one remains always hesitant, and 'the problems of the neuronal basis of consciousness will not be resolved for a very long time' [516].

2. PSYCHOLOGICAL ANALGESIA

Psychological analgesia can be studied experimentally by means of hypnotically-produced analgesia. The influence, via speech, of one individual on another can effectively produce an analgesia. Wolff and Goodell have been able to show experimentally that the threshold of pain varies under the effect of suggestion: for instance, taking a placebo as an analgesic raises the threshold for pain, whilst it is lowered if the patient is informed that he has in fact taken bicarbonate. The psychophysiological mechanism of analgesia produced by psychotherapy, whether under hypnosis or in the waking state, is fundamentally the same. In both cases it consists of a blocking, or rather of a central modification of pain perception through the intervention of affective factors. In hypnosis this modification operates, so to speak, on a macroscopic scale. But we still remain ignorant of the essential mechanisms of these phenomena both physiological and psychological, and the relationships between the two are still far from having been elucidated. Researches are being carried out mainly along two lines. They attempt to answer two questions: *how* and *why* does speech have an analgesic action? Both the mechanism and the motivation must be explained.

The Russians explain the '*how*' in terms of cortical excitation and inhibition, corresponding at the psychological level to the well-known phenomenon of attention. The way in which speech works, according to Pavlov (cf. p. 102), is as a stimulus which itself is just as material as any other physical stimulus. In studying the language of the hypnotist (which represents an exaggeration of all verbal action), Pavlov writes 'the words of the hypnotist constitute an excitation, this excitation, in the presence of a certain degree of cortical inhibition which spreads, then becomes concentrated in a single channel following the general law of excitation; at the same time it provokes a profound, indirect inhibition in the remainder of the cortex, and through that itself excludes any action, and competes with other traces of excitation, present and past'.

This conception of a purely cortical mechanism of inhibition is criticized today. For instance, DELL and BONVALLET [122] consider that 'it is difficult today to accept the notion of an inhibition which spreads by a purely cortical mechanism, just as it is difficult to imagine a precise mechanism which corresponds to terms such as excitation, inhibition, irradiation and concentration which have been used in conditioned reflexology'. Whilst on this subject, it must be pointed out that thanks to progress in electrophysiology and to research into the reticular system, attempts have now been made which may allow the objectivation of the neurophysiological mechanisms of attention and inhibition in animals [236, 237, 259, 214, 229]. But in man, individual variations in reactivity to speech exist. This is the problem of the 'why'. The Pavlovian school reply to this question as follows: if speech produces an effect on one individual and not on another, then that is due to the peculiarities of his Nervous Type.

The concept of Nervous Types (cf. pp. 112, 136), which has been studied chiefly in animals, presents difficulties when it is transposed to man. In man it is made up, not only of the inborn but of the acquired as well, by the biological just as much as the social, encompassing the phenomena of learning used in its broadest sense. This underlines the need to understand the whole of a person's past history. It is only by so doing that one can understand why a particular word can have a pain-reducing action on one individual and not on another.

But the past history contains the memories of both conscious and unconscious events. Russian authors have not taken into account any but the first, and it is just because of this that the Pavlovian concept of Nervous Types is so limited, dealing as it does only with the more superficial layers of the personality. Unconscious motivation still remains, and this may be important in allowing us to understand the analgesia which results from the verbal action exercised by one individual on another in an interpersonal relationship. This latter, whether it is based upon hypnosis, or the more ordinary doctor–patient relationship, involves an emotional factor.

The psychoanalytic school has studied this emotional relationship in putting forward the idea of transference. By this latter term is understood, according to Lagache 'in the course of psychoanalytic treatment a complex attitude develops on the part of the analysand *vis-à-vis* the analyst, in particular affective reactions, either hostile or more generally ambivalent (a positive or negative transference); these attitudes instead of being responses arising out of the actual situation, reflect residual conflicts with persons in the child's environment'.

Thus, through the introduction of the idea of transference, having recognized the importance of unconscious motivations in an interpersonal relationship, the psychoanalysts have nevertheless not as yet defined the kind of motivations which are found in psychologically produced analgesia. It is well known that affectivity modifies the threshold of pain perception, but the precise mechanism for this modification is not known. The blocking of painful perception by psychological procedures, based on emotional motivations, can operate in very different ways, the integration taking place at different levels. This modification is not made in a vertical manner, by a variation of the intensity, as we will see in reporting clinical observations. Again, considering only obstetrical matters, it will be remembered that previous observations have been made on women who were delivered in a somnambulistic state. For instance, about 1860, Liébault, and later other clinicians, both in France and elsewhere at different periods, had noted different types of hypnotic analgesia. The parturient women themselves declared that they felt the contractions, but that they were not painful; others said that they felt a pain but did not suffer. 'Here comes a bad pain, doctor, here comes a little pain' said one woman to Dumontpallier when she was in a somnambulistic state. Still others, under hypnosis, manifest motor and vegetative signs of suffering, whilst in fact maintaining that they did not suffer. Again, some women on waking up have forgotten the pain and the whole event.

In the light of these experiences, the varieties of patterns of experience of pain perception can be seen to be numerous. A century later (1950) in a discussion (organized by the Josiah Macy Foundation in New York) on 'The perception of pain and some factors which modify it,' the same problem was again brought up without any satisfactory explanation being made. BRENMAN [60] described similar attitudes to those which have just been described, in women who were delivered under hypnosis.

Some said 'I do have pain, but it does not bother me'. Others maintained that they did not suffer at all, while presenting all the external signs of pain. Still others had forgotten the whole childbirth, whether they had shown signs of suffering or not. She states that there is still no explanation for these different forms of pain perception. The first appears to her the most baffling. She tentatively put forward a hypothesis linking the ideas of transference and of attention. 'Attention,' she said, 'if we can use that undefined concept here, was directed to whatever the physician was doing and was so gratifying that possibly then the experience of pain was not so important any longer'. In the same discussion, FROMM-REICHMANN [183] reported that Marsh, Moore and Vollmer of San Francisco, obstetricians with a psychoanalytic outlook, were allowing their women in labour to observe in a mirror the course of their delivery. They did not suffer. Fromm-Reichmann herself put forward the hypothesis that the attention of parturient women was concentrated on a process whose emotional significance was more important than the pain.

During the same meeting RAPAPORT [452], the author of the book *Emotions and Memory*, stressed that 'the attention mechanism would not be a question of a certain amount of attention shifted from one place to another . . . but a matter of complex dynamics and not a simple shift of quantity. We deal here with qualitative changes and multiple dimensions'. It should be added that analgesia can be obtained by posthypnotic suggestion, which again implies a phenomenon concerned with memory, and whose relationships with affectivity are quite clear but complex; the neurophysiological mechanisms of memory are absolutely unknown.

In conclusion, if verbally-produced analgesia or psychotherapeutically produced analgesia is a well established experimental fact, it is important to recognise that the physiological and psychological mechanisms are as yet very imperfectly understood.

3. THE 'NATURAL' CHARACTER OF THE PAIN OF CHILDBIRTH

The problem of the nature of the pain of childbirth is very controversial. Read (p. 53) and Velvovski (p. 102) postulate that pain is not an inherent part of the physiological process of childbirth. With both it partakes of elements acquired under the influence of sociocultural and emotional factors. For Velvovski the pain appears in the local changes or central neurodynamic changes. As we have already seen, his ideas are disputed by the majority of writers, who, whilst recognizing the importance of reflex conditional and emotional factors which can increase the pain, nevertheless consider that the pain of childbirth is a normal phenomenon. Animals suffer, a phylogenetic finality is even assigned to this suffering, and on the other hand the act of childbirth by its exceptional character cannot be absolutely compared to other physiological phenomena. In order to establish their hypothesis, Velvovski and Read underline the fact that (a) in civilized societies, some women go through childbirth naturally without pain and that (b) in certain primitive societies, this is the general rule. These arguments will be considered in greater detail.

(a) Painless Childbirth in a Civilized Society

It is well known that in our society, a certain percentage of women, from 7 to 14 per cent according to Velvovski, who have no anatomical peculiarity, have a painless childbirth. The explanation of this is difficult. It could be perhaps interpreted in two different ways, either that these women ought to be considered as normal, and the other 90 per cent present anomalies, either somatic or psychological; or on the other hand, that pain is the rule and analgesia is the result of structural peculiarities. These may be situated probably either on a purely neurological level, and bring about a natural analgesia, or at a psychological level, in which case there would be an absence of 'negative' emotions, or the presence of 'positive' emotions, such as the joy of maternity, which might cover up the negative emotions.

It would be interesting to define the different aspects of the personalities of those women who have a painless childbirth; for instance it is known that the capacity for obtaining a deep hypnotic state with anaesthesia is found in approximately the same proportion of patients. Would not the women who are naturally analgesic and those who constitute the group of complete successes with preparation also fall into the latter group? The study of their suggestibility would perhaps enable us to answer the question. The understanding of their individual characteristics would at the same time help us to establish criteria of predictibility regarding the efficacy of such or such a method in its application to other pregnant women.

(b) *Childbirth in Primitive Societies*

It is certain that variations in resistance to pain do occur, although it is difficult to say whether they arise from variations in the intensity of the pain, properly speaking, or in the expression of the pain. HADDON [213] in 1907 observed a resistance to pain in certain primitive people which is inconceivable amongst Occidentals, and TERRY [524] has described tribes who are able to endure burns without apparent pain. As to the pain of childbirth very few ethnological studies exist; usually the problem is mentioned in the course of more general ethnological work. Care must be exercised because it is possible that in certain peoples the woman does not express pain, but this does not mean that she does not suffer. HRDLICKA [235], for instance, has reported that Mohave Indian women undoubtedly suffer in the course of their childbirth, but the expression of their suffering is held back through fear of ridicule. PREISSMAN and OGOULBOSTAN-ESSENOVA [434] (Achkhabad) reported that Turkmenian women behave calmly during childbirth but this does not mean that they do not feel it as painful, if one judges the matter according to the women's own statements. Childbirth is considered by these women as a job to be got through. The writers believe that this is the result of customs 'whose roots are found in a secular tradition amongst Turkmenian women of childbirth without making a sound, in a disciplined way'. Custom decrees that the women are delivered outside the house in the absence of any strange person and even if they do suffer they must dissimulate any motor expression of their suffering. Those women, who are delivered nowadays in maternity hospitals, still preserve the same behaviour.

MARGARET MEAD [359] attaches importance to sociocultural influences on the expression of the pain of childbirth. 'Childbirth may be experienced according to the phrasing given it by the culture, as an experience that is dangerous and painful, interesting and engrossing, matter-of-fact and mildly hazardous or accompanied by enormous supernatural hazards'. Pregnancy is

AN EXAMINATION OF THE PROBLEMS

not always considered as beneficial: it can be felt to be dangerous, as with the Aztecs. Margaret Mead also brings up the problem of the male contribution to the patterning of the experience of pregnancy and childbirth. 'There seems some reason to believe', she says, 'that male imagination, undisciplined and uninformed by immediate bodily clues or immediate bodily experience, may have contributed disproportionately to the cultural superstructure of belief and practice regarding childbearing'.

Opposing the view that deliveries would be easier in primitive peoples, Jochelson thinks that among the Yakuts and Youkaghirs, where women have to rapidly resume their occupations, they suffer chronic disorders, nervous exhaustion and early senescence.

FORD [165] has studied the literature concerning reproduction in 64 primitive societies. As far as the pain of childbirth is concerned, he writes 'the popular impression of childbirth in primitive society as painless and easy is definitely contradicted by our cases. As a matter of fact it is often both prolonged and painful. Fear of a difficult and painful labour motivates women in all societies to follow strict rules during pregnancy'. Moreover, the majority of these tribes have recourse to special techniques in cases where the childbirth might be particularly difficult. FREEDMAN and FERGUSON [172], reviewing the different works bearing on painless childbirth amongst primitives, consider that pain is always present; while in some tribes it does appear that painful reactions are generally less frequent than among us, the overwhelming majority have pain comparable to ours, and in not a few others it appears even more frequently and dramatically'.* Therapeutic procedures which facilitate the childbirth are found amongst all these peoples. The Maoris of New Zealand play on the flute, the Yakoutes employ Shamans who have the function of driving out the evil spirits which have made the woman ill.

These writers also drew attention to the fact that tenderness is not always associated with pregnancy. Amongst the Samoyedes, for instance, pregnancy is considered to be despicable; amongst

---

*Ethnological observations do not mention if these deliveries were dystocic, or normal but painful. It is therefore impossible to know if the therapeutic procedure was aimed at the physiology of delivery or at pain itself. One may wonder whether these two phenomena are distinguished in the mind of the primitive.

the Ashanti it is shameful to die in child-bed.* Freedman and Ferguson deduce, quite in contrast to the views of Read, that pain is not a product of civilization, which in itself brings about an emotional instability. If this were in fact the case, in societies which have the most emotional stability, more painless childbirths would occur.

Inversely, groups with sexual repressions and intense inhibitions ought to have more difficult labours; but in fact this is not always the case. Conditioning by the environment has only a partial influence on the pain of childbirth. Comparable patterns of reaction to the pain can be found in quite dissimilar civilizations. For instance, in Samoa, the natives are stable, and have apparently easy labours, but in fact, the expression of pain is forbidden. Without this inhibition, the reaction to the pain would doubtless appear. As opposed to this fact the Cuna women, who have the most powerful prohibitions, do not have deliveries which would differ from those of Samoan women. On the whole, Freedman and Ferguson conclude that against the background of an undeniably physiological substrate, pain can be increased by cultural factors or by individual stresses.

Concerning therapeutic procedures used by primitive peoples, we shall report the analysis made by Levi-Strauss of a ritual which was collected and published by the Swedish ethnologists Holmer and Wassen. This ritual, practised by the Cuna Indians of Panama in difficult deliveries, consists of a chant, sung by a tribal medicine man. Levi-Strauss compares this shamanistic cure to a psychological treatment based on psychodynamic concepts analagous to psychoanalysis among civilized peoples: no manipulation of the body, no drugs, only speech is used. Since the physiological disorder is caused by psychological and social motivations, it must be repaired in the same way. According to

*In our culture, on the contrary, motherhood is valued. In certain populations, it is considered a blessing. A German doctor, GRASSL [205] who practised for many years among very devout Bavarian peasants, reports that they consider motherhood a gift of God. They think that a woman who dies during childbirth is cleansed of all her sins and goes straight to Heaven; she is dressed in white and carried to the churchyard by young girls also clad in white. Grassl adds that, in difficult deliveries, he has called in a priest, who exerted a very relaxing influence on the woman.

AN EXAMINATION OF THE PROBLEMS

Levi-Strauss, the therapist, an incarnation of authority, has as his aim, 'to translate into a language meaningful for the patient, thus enabling him to name and to understand, possibly also to dominate pains which were prior to that impossible to express, in their real and figurative meaning'.

These ethnological studies show that childbirth is a painful phenomenon in all primitive societies. It can of course be maintained that these societies are already very far from that state of nature which the proponents of this theory seem to envisage, but that is a question that cannot be debated here.

(c) Parturition in Animals

RIVIÈRE and CHASTRUSSE [468] of Bordeaux studied this subject with regard to domestic animals. They write: 'It does not seem that veterinarians are unanimous in their interpretations of the manifestations which have been observed in parturient animals. Some would consider the period of dilatation in the Bovidae as painless; the animal continues in its usual habits without appearing to be disturbed by the pain. At the time of delivery, on the contrary, it stops grazing, becomes agitated and restless throughout the contraction. This restlessness may be the expression of pain, in the way we understand it, or may be simply a feeling of malaise or of something strange; it is clearly impossible to decide which. Other veterinarians are much more definite in their views. For instance, parturition amongst large domestic animals such as cows and mares is clearly painful. Beginning at the period of dilatation, the animal separates itself from the rest of the herd, lies down, gets up, while its flanks heave restlessly. At the moment of delivery the pains become much more acute, the animal groans and cries, demonstrating by its expression a very obvious suffering. Epidural anaesthesia, systematically practised for all intrauterine interventions, has an immediate effect in bringing about a cessation of these manifestations; the animal begins to graze again, even during the operative intervention.

'The bitch also very clearly manifests pain in the course of parturition. Behaviour varies with the different species and, above all, with the conditions in which the animal has been brought up. Bitches which have been brought up a little hardily, such as foxhounds or greyhounds, seem to be fairly well able to endure the uterine contractions. Bitches-*de-luxe*, however, often brought up by women, make a great deal of noise with the pains which are felt at the time of the uterine contractions, and above all, at the moment when the puppy is expelled. Small laboratory animals, such as rats, mice, guinea pigs and rabbits do not appear to show pain at the moment of their delivery. It seems then that the higher the animal on the scale of species* and the more (in a particular species) it has been made the object of particular care, then the more the sensations felt during the uterine contractions will be exteriorized'.

M. Jacques Nouvel, Professor at the Musée de l'Homme and Director of the Zoological Garden in Paris, has very kindly given us his opinion concerning pain felt by wild animals in captivity during their delivery. He considers that there is little difference between wild animals in captivity and domestic animals in their behaviour during parturition. In one as in the other, when a lesion occurs, which in man would be painful, the resulting behaviour can have a most pernicious effect. For instance, self-mutilation by a carnivore with a fractured leg, or the production of a cutaneous lesion owing to pruritus or the presence of a surgical scar may both occur. Nouvel has never observed such happenings during delivery, but on the contrary, only behaviour which favours its accomplishment.

It seems then that even if birth is painful, the sensation which accompanies this physiological event is insufficiently intense to alter behaviour. There are no studies of parturition amongst wild beasts in their natural conditions. M. F. Lagneau, Professor of the Pathology of Reproduction at the Veterinary School of Maison-Alfort, has drawn our attention to some facts relating to parturition in animals. Behaviour during delivery varies according to species. It is, for instance, more disorganized with the mare than with the cow; parturition is more difficult amongst half-bred than pure-bred strains. Younger animals have more difficulty than their elders—this equally applies to primiparae as to multiparae. The individual differences when they concern the same species are insignificant. Parturition is easier and more rapid

---

*It is a mistake to assume that certain rodents (rats for instance) are phylogenetically inferior to the Bovidae.

amongst females having multiple offspring, owing to the small size of the foetus.

Michel Fontaine at Alfort Veterinary School was kind enough to communicate the following facts: he believes that two periods must be distinguished in delivery: that of contractions prior to mobilization of the foetus, and that of the passage of the newborn animal into the pelvis. He does not consider that the first is painful, and is shown only by signs of unrest or of preoccupations which are more or less expressive according to the species (more disorderly in horses and nervous small dogs, quieter in bovines...); it is possible at that period to dissociate defence reactions to induced pain from the reactions to uterine contractions. There is moreover a change in the respiratory movements, which are quicker and less deep. When the foetus is expelled pain is more obvious if the passage is more difficult. It seems related to compression exerted on the pelvic walls.

Certain veterinarians believe that the atmosphere of the stable, and even the affection which is manifested in the attitude of the people around can influence the behaviour of the female parturient. ELIGULACHVILI [145] in his study on gestation and parturition in apes, has pointed out that suffering does not show itself by cries and groans; even in cases of bony fracture they remain silent. But, this author adds, there is undoubtedly suffering in the course of the delivery, and it is shown by restlessness and contortions.

4. EMOTIONAL FACTORS AND THE PAIN OF CHILDBIRTH

The two schools, the English and the Russian, assign an important role to emotional factors in the genesis of the pain of childbirth. Read gives an essential role to the fear; the Russians, however, consider that the fear, whilst it does not play an essential role, has nevertheless an undeniable effect. It has not been proved that fear can provoke pain, but it is probable that it can influence pain sensibility. One cannot, however, foresee in which way. For instance, it is known that terror experienced during a fight can produce an analgesia. Chlifer, as we have seen, reported a case of analgesia in a woman threatened by the death sentence [92].

As to pain in childbirth, the significance of the word 'fear' must be considered. Conscious fears are not the most important. They often cover deeper unconscious fears which simple rational persuasion has no chance of making disappear. Amongst others, the Russian Plotitcher (cf. p. 119), who has studied the fear of childbirth tells us that frequently the fear is 'irrational'; it seems to be more connected with anxiety* than with fear, although the delimitation may not always be very clear. In these conditions we are led to examine the relationship of anxiety to pain in general, and in particular to the pain of childbirth.

(a) *Anxiety and Pain*

Studies on pain in the psychoanalytic literature are very uncommon. Freud himself admitted that this was a very obscure region of mental life. In 1920 in *Beyond the Pleasure Principle* he wrote:

'We would readily express our gratitude to any philosophical or psychological theory which was able to inform us of the meaning of the feelings of pleasure and unpleasure which act so imperatively upon us. But on this point we are, alas, offered nothing to our purpose. This is the most obscure and inaccessible region of the mind, and, since we cannot avoid contact with it, the least rigid hypothesis, it seems to me, will be the best.

'We have decided to relate pleasure and unpleasure to the quantity of excitation that is present in the mind but is not in any way "bound" and to relate them in such a manner that unpleasure corresponds to an increase in the quantity of excitation and pleasure to a diminution' [178].

In fact the term 'pain' (Unlust)† is in more general use, encompassing all types of pain, whether psychological or physical. Freud

*GRINKER [205] who has thoroughly studied the problem of anxiety from the psychosomatic point of view stresses the complexity of research in this field. The concept of unconscious anxiety does not lend itself to the establishment of fruitful psychosomatic hypotheses because we cannot consider a person to be anxious unless he consciously experiences this unbearable feeling and whatever idiosyncratic accompaniments it provokes.'

†In German 'Unlust' (displeasure) is translated as pain with inverted commas and 'schmerz' as pain without inverted commas.

AN EXAMINATION OF THE PROBLEMS

rarely speaks of physical pain in a specific manner. 'Probably', he wrote, 'the specific discomfort of bodily pain is the result of some local breaking through of the barrier against stimuli. From this point in the periphery there streams to the central psychic apparatus continual excitation such as would otherwise come only from within'. In 1926 he took up the problem again in his book *Inhibitions, Symptoms and Anxiety*. 'We still know very little concerning pain', he wrote. He tried to formulate the relationships between anxiety, pain and mourning. SCHILDER [492] has studied these pain phenomena in their relationships with the modifications of the body image. SZASZ [520] who has recently made an up-to-date survey of the problem remarks that there is a surprising lack of psychoanalytic contributions to the problem of pain, and himself attempts to formulate the relationships between anxiety and pain in connection with *object relationship*. He postulates a stage of undifferentiation between anxiety and pain in infants before the age of four months. There exists a single affect, anxiety-pain. Then between from four to nine months it is differentiated into pain (in relation to the body) and anxiety (in relation to objects): 'Pain, as an affect warning the ego of possible injury or loss of the body, is a construct analogous to anxiety as a signal warning the ego of the danger of (interpersonal) object loss'. Szasz remarks that these affects can be used as defences, one against the other. Certain personalities, for instance, hysterics, will utilize pain as a defence against anxiety, others, particularly rather rigid personalities, will use this mechanism the other way round.

(b) *Anxiety and the Pain of Childbirth*

The relationships between anxiety and the pain of childbirth are still very poorly understood. It is clear that pregnancy and delivery are events of the first importance in the woman's emotional life. Not only do positive emotions make their appearance, but old anxieties, until then dormant, can be activated in the course of the pregnancy. It is not unusual to see neurosis beginning or being exacerbated after childbirth.

BLOOS [47] of Huntington, U.S.A. gives a clinical description of the justifiable and non-justifiable fears felt by pregnant women. In the first group he includes fears of syphilis, diabetes, heart disease, and tuberculosis, whilst the second group he explains as resulting from ideas of losing her figure, of not pleasing her husband, of being deformed by breast feeding, of having a deformed child or of dying during the childbirth.

PLOTITCHER [430], using a simple questionnaire, has found fears present in 83 per cent of pregnant women, KATCHAN and BELOZERSKI in 71 per cent. HELEN DEUTSCH [126] herself considers that in all women, the happy and the disappointed, the strong and the weak, the loving and the hating—the doubts, restlessness, impatience, and joyful expectations all conceal the fear of delivery, which is increasingly intensified with the approach of term.

What is the origin of these fears? Read and Velvovski consider them as sociocultural in origin. The beliefs are anchored in the ineluctable character of the pain of childbirth and transmitted by one generation to the other, by word of mouth, and by the written word. The original fears have arisen, according to Velvovski, from very painful pathological childbirth in the distant past due to the lack of hygiene, and through marriages being made at a very early age.*

In her book *The Psychology of Women*, Deutsch has studied these fears psychoanalytically, as well as other psychological problems linked with pregnancy and childbirth. She recognizes that real dangers do exist, even in the most normal conditions, due to factors such as pain, haemorrhages, etc. Moreover, reality factors, both economic and social, can produce anxiety. But even when the real danger is eliminated fear exists, because, she says, 'we assume that all these fears are only provocations or intensifications of a deep hereditary fear of death that accompanies a new life awakening in the mother's body'. This fear is overdetermined, one of its principal aspects being the fear of separation from the child, with whom the mother identifies herself in living again the traumatism of her own birth.† This separation is also linked to infantile fears bearing on excretory and retentive

---

*Here there seems to be a contradiction. On the one hand Velvovski evokes, as well as Read, a Golden Age, and on the other hand speaks of a large number of painful childbirths in the first years of humanity. Recent studies on primitive people, show, amongst other things, that the primitive woman is no more favourably placed than her civilized sister.

†Cf. Rank's book *Birth Trauma* [449].

functions. Childbirth can flare up old anxieties. 'Childbirth reawakes the psychic contents which have accompanied the excretory processes at different periods of life. The process of being born, by its actual resemblance to intestinal movements can reawake a previous situation and the emotions which accompanied it'. Moreover, 'another source of the fear of death in childbirth resides in the relationship of the woman with her mother, an unresolved and guilt-laden relationship'.*

Other writers have tried to confirm these hypotheses of Helen Deutsch by a study of pregnant women from the psychoanalytic point of view. KLEIN et al. [269] studied 27 primiparae during pregnancy and labour, and produced evidence of the anxiety provoking factors studied by Helen Deutsch. Emotional difficulties in existence at the time of the pregnancy became magnified in the course of pregnancy. They confirmed the identification of the pregnant woman with her mother; in cases where their mothers had had a difficult delivery the same difficulties were likely in the daughter.† FODOR [162], using the dreams of pregnant women, again insists on the identification of the mother with the child, and on the memory of the anxiety of birth.

Having discussed the existence of anxiety linked with pregnancy and childbirth we can now pass to its relationship with the pain. According to Helen Deutsch anxiety linked with the act of childbirth underlines a masochistic regressive attitude *vis-à-vis* the suffering brought about by childbirth. The pregnant woman in her reactions to the pain and anxiety, according to the predominant aspect of her personality will retreat into passivity or an untimely activity. The conflict between the active and

*Thus the presence of the midwife during the birth satisfies not only the need for comfort from a kindly person, but can have deeper unconscious meanings. The doctor's presence also comes into play at several different levels.

†We have experienced exactly the opposite in a case where the mother of the parturient had had a very painful, restless and disturbed delivery. The daughter consciously refused to identify with her mother and after the most minimal preparation went through labour in a most calm and well-behaved manner. HACK TUKE [543] reported an observation, made by Laycock (1840) in which the mother identified herself with her parturient daughter. Childbirth was very painful and the 48-year-old woman, menopausal eight years previously, showed strong 'uterine contractions'. Three days later she secreted milk.

passive tendencies can be expressed in physical phenomena and can influence the quality of the labour and the pain. The question of the relationships between anxiety and pain has also been examined by GREENACRE [202] in her paper on the 'Biological economy of birth'. For her, pain has a self-protective value; 'it resembles in this respect anxiety, the signal of hidden (future or inner) danger and fear, the reaction to outer danger. Indeed in some states pain, anxiety and fear are not readily distinguishable one from another, and in a larger sense all are varieties of pain, if we consider this as a distress, the opposite of pleasure.' FREEDMAN et al. [173] consider this a useful concept. Throughout their study of memory processes in the pregnant woman, they remark on the different ways in which the fear, the anxiety and the pain are remembered; 'Our mothers recall pain; they also recall fear, that is, a relatively focused response to an external danger. However, anxiety—by which we mean a state of apprehension arising primarily from internal motivational and adaptational conflict which is characterized by an inability to act—is more prone to amnestic and paramnestic changes'.

KARTCHNER [261] of Salt Lake City (U.S.A.) has studied the emotional reactions to childbirth in 500 women who had received no preparation. They were questioned before and after the birth, and observed during delivery. He acknowledges the relative value of such a study owing to the subjectivity of the material, as well as that of the observer. He believes that consciously felt fears represent only one aspect of the problem; nevertheless, his figures showed that fear and anxiety augment disagreeable sensations, both emotional and physical, and owing to this the number of difficult deliveries are increased. In spite of more than half of the women experiencing fears of different kinds, 85 per cent of them had had a satisfying labour.

STRAKER [513] of Montreal studied 13 pregnant women who were neurotic, and having psychotherapy at the time of their pregnancy and childbirth. In spite of the presence of a considerable degree of anxiety, he states that their labours were astonishingly short, easy and calm, and that they collaborated cheerfully with the doctor. The women themselves were amazed at this. He attributes the ease of childbirth in these women to the influence of psychotherapy with an important psychological preparation for childbirth. This preparation consisted of 'anticipating the details of the experience and exploring their fears and attitudes, utilizing corrective reassurance and education, etc. . . .'

KUBIE [289], discussing the work of Davidson, believes that 'the effect of anxiety on pain as a human experience is a physiologic as well as a psychologic reality. Many examples of this have long been known with regard to pain which has its origin in the gastrointestinal tract, in the bladder and in mutilations'. The educational process,* Kubie believes, 'lessens the normal anxiety of the more normal prospective mother and thus reduces both the fear and the impact of pain . . . presumably it reduces the involuntary perineal spasms'.

Faced with the complexity of the relationship between anxiety and the pain of childbirth, some psychosomatic hypotheses may be tentatively formulated. Emotional factors in the pain of childbirth occur at two levels; at the physiological level they can produce localized somatic effects, such as spasms, and at the central level an emotion intensifies pain perception (pain, it is known, can even exist in the absence of peripheral stimuli). On the whole most writers have envisaged two levels of pain in childbirth. Read speaks of a 'true pain' and of a 'false pain'; Velvovski postulates a somatic pain, due to a local pathology, and a central pain due to a central neurodynamic disturbance. Nicolaiev, Konstantinov and others, adhere to the notion of two levels of pain, but criticize Velvovski, mainly for underestimating the local physiological factor in pain (Velvovski and Read agree in considering the pain of childbirth as pathological).

But these writers have not considered that the same emotional events can give rise to both types of pain (in the sense of their increase or even of their origin). These emotional happenings sometimes act directly at the level of a local somatic change, sometimes at the level of central perception. The question of whether the pain of childbirth is physiological or pathological will not be discussed here; the majority of authors contradict Read and Velvovski, and maintain that it is physiological. The psychological action, as applied to emotional factors, can be effective at two levels, locally, in eliminating the emotional cause (anxiety) which is the base of the somatic disturbance (spasm), and at the central perceptive level, by eliminating the emotional tension. In both cases, this action has taken place by eliminating the cause of the pain. It could then be said that it takes on a prophylactic character. But psychological action is not confined to the elimination of the cause of the pain, it can equally abolish or modify all pain perception, as is shown by our experience of hypnotic analgesia.

*Later we shall see the limits which the author assigns to education.

The action can thus be therapeutic. It is not always possible in practice to distinguish clearly the two levels of psychological action.

5. PSYCHOLOGICAL ANALGESIA IN OBSTETRICS

The theoretical concepts of psychologically produced analgesia are poorly understood. Hypnotically produced analgesia still provides an experimental basis for its study. In order to judge the efficacy of the procedures employed in these methods of psychologically produced obstetrical analgesia criteria are unhappily lacking. In the hypnosuggestive method the mode of action rests essentially on hypnotic suggestion. What then are the analgesiant factors in the methods of Read and of Velvovski and what is their respective role? Three can be distinguished: (a) the didactic factor, (b) the physiotherapeutic factor, and (c) the psychotherapeutic factor. These three factors are only separated for convenience, in reality they are closely interconnected.

(a) The Didactic Factor

It is well known that information can have a beneficial effect. It familiarizes the woman with the anatomy and physiology of childbirth, thus combating the unknown—one of the causes of fear. In psychoanalytic language we could say that it operates as DONOVAN and LANDISBERG [133] stress, by the substitution of facts for phantasy.* Kubie believes, concerning 'educated childbirth', that 'the severity of the impact of pain, whether as an imminent threat or as a current reality, can be lessened if anxiety and its attendant phantasies (both conscious and unconscious) can be diminished'. This anxiety can be diminished in part 'through vivid and frank education as to the nature of the body, its normal function, its resilience, and also its vulnerability. In other words, by diminishing the mystery of the body one can usually diminish its terror'.

We believe that teaching is equally important at the social level, by raising the level of education and also at the individual level, by increasing the potentialities of the personality and the possibility of mastery (reinforcement of the ego). Moreover, the

*It is understood that the problem is much more complex. There are phantasies which are not reducible by simple information.

didactic element brings the woman into a personal relationship with the person preparing her, and with the members of a group, itself of psychotherapeutic importance. Understanding alone does not suffice to produce an analgesia. The proof is that women doctors and midwives, as Konstantinov rightly emphasized at the Kiev Congress, can have a painful childbirth, in spite of their knowledge of the processes at work. Kubie also draws attention to the limits of education. '. . . There is a specific limit to the extent to which anxiety can be diminished through such education alone. This limit is set at the boundary of neurosis . . . where unconscious and distorted sources of anxiety enter the picture, educational processes alone must always fail. The reason for this is obvious, namely that unconscious psychological processes are not accessible to education, any more than they are accessible to rewards and punishments, to arguments or appeals to reason, to exhortation or threats.'

(b) *The Physiotherapeutic Factor**

This comprises essentially the physical, respiratory, and relaxation exercises.

(1) *Physical Exercises*

By this we mean the particular movements involved in physical training, not including respiratory exercises and muscular relaxation. Physical exercises are useful for the general physical and mental condition, but do not produce an analgesia proper; women who are very athletic do not spontaneously have any the less painful childbirth. NOTTER and EGRON [403] report that Hans Guggisberg considers that some sports, such as equitation, or ski-ing can produce an excessively muscular perineum.

*NIXON [398] believes that physiotherapy has a psychosomatic action. This is how he expresses it: 'the mind–body partnership can sometimes be approached more effectively through bodily action than through complicated mental processes.

'It is part of an attitude toward the body which is one of the chief contributions of people like the physiotherapists, whose approach to their patient's "mind–body" entity is through helping her to understand her body, control it, use it, establish friendly relations with it, to regard it as a creature with which they can work happily, and which is neither to be allowed free rein nor yet driven on the curb.'

They themselves have recorded 'some observations concerning long and painful labour in teachers of gymnastics'.

However, Laszlo, Gyula and Laszlo consider that intensive gymnastics, under the direction of trained personnel, do not harm the woman's body, but favour the course of childbirth. They studied 140 women who had practised intensive gymnastics for at least three years. In 87·2 per cent of them, delivery was twice as rapid as in non-athletic women. There were only two per cent of Caesarean sections, and six per cent of forceps applications.

Nicolaiev also recently stressed the advantages of gymnastics in pregnant women. 'Gymnastics', he says, 'have a beneficial action on various organs and primarily on the brain'. [392].

(2) *Respiratory Exercises*

Their effect has been interpreted in different ways. In the Psychoprophylactic Method, as practised in the Soviet Union, respiratory exercises are considered as processes which reduce pain by distracting attention, an empirical measure which has been known for many years. The general explanation put forward by the Pavlovian School is that a focus of excitation is produced by means of attention, and that inhibitory phenomena accompany it. Velvovski's new hypothesis, according to which an elevation of threshold by excitation is produced, has so far not been proved. Plotitcher believes that both solutions are acceptable.

Respiratory exercises, for Read's School, have a local physiological value (increased suggestion) as well as a more general relaxatory value, but their mode of action is not clearly defined. Prill deals with respiration in a more detailed manner. He assigns importance both to oxygenation, and to the respiratory rhythm itself in obtaining total relaxation. Moreover, we believe, the focusing of attention on the respiratory mechanism has a pain reducing effect in a similar way to that claimed by the Russians.

It is clear that there is a relation between respiration and the emotional states which find their expression via the respiratory system. Respiratory factors are important in Yoga, and the Yogis themselves are able to produce complete anaesthesia.

(3) *Relaxation*

The problem of relaxation is most complex, the term itself frequently leading to confusion. The two principal techniques which have been used, those of Schultz and of Jacobson, demand a very specialized knowledge and cannot be applied in obstetrical analgesia except on a very limited scale. For SCHULTZ [497, 498] (p. 82) relaxation is an active process of concentration, it is one of the constituent elements of hypnotic states, whilst JACOBSON [245, 246] (p. 81) considers that hypnosis implies tension whereas relaxation is a passive process of 'letting go'.

Read's adherents favour Jacobson's technique, but carry it out only in a very approximate manner, so that Jacobson criticizes the use which has been made of his method. On the other hand American authors, such as Kroger and Mandy, using the hypnosuggestive method, believe that relaxation exercises often produce hypnoid states. Analgesia can be the product of the suggestibility inherent in these states. Certain doctors, to improve their results, go further, and from relaxation and a hypnoid state pass directly to hypnosis itself (ABRAMSON and HERON [2] and MICHAEL [366]).

The French proponents of the Psychoprophylactic Method practice relaxation in a manner very much resembling that of Read under the name of neuromuscular education or muscular release. The Russians consider relaxation is one of the first hypnotic manifestations, and according to their terminology, is therefore a state of inhibition. At the time when Velvovski emphasized the prophylactic value of 'excitation' or of 'activation', in contradistinction to 'inhibition' which possessed a therapeutic role, relaxation tended to fall into disuse. Inasmuch as it was an inhibitory procedure it was reserved for pathological childbirths. In fact Plotitcher in 1954 recommended 'relaxing-rest' or the hypnoid state for pathological childbirths, advising the practice of muscular release between the contractions, without insisting on the production of hypnoid states. At the Kiev Conference in 1956 NOCOLAIEV [393] recommended a training in muscular release.

As to the carrying out of the exercises, and the eventual transition to hypnoid states we believe that individual differences exist. Moreover, even when such states are produced, they represent a positive phenomenon. In Pavlovian terms these phasic states signify an increase of suggestibility and constitute an immediate or delayed analgesic factor. In analytic terms one could speak of a regression being able to modify pain sensibility by virtue of the emotional relationship with the therapist.

The question of the *active* or *passive* attitude of the pregnant woman during childbirth is difficult to evaluate. She can combine an active attitude toward the total act of childbirth with a transient passivity aimed at raising the threshold of pain, but this passivity which itself reduces pain is considered by some as an active process. Schultz speaks of a 'concentrative' decontraction, his disciple Prill of 'concentrated passivity'. The anaesthesia that is found among Yogis seems to rest on the active mechanism of attention, and this has been shown by some authors through electrophysiological means [98]. How to assess in what degree the woman should combine activity and passivity is a question which will depend on her personality. It would be useful here to have some criteria of predictability.

The personality of the woman must also be considered in order to define her attitude in regard to relaxation. Certain women use relaxation as a relational experience and will adopt a passive attitude, almost going to sleep in the course of the exercises. The analgesiant benefit to them will be felt later on (as in post-hypnotic suggestion)—others prepared by the same technique will find in relaxation a means of concentrating their attention, giving proof of their activity and will benefit from it during the delivery itself (pain-reducing procedure).

It is only by mentioning these views that we can see our way clear to reconciling the apparently different opinions with regard to the nature of relaxation.

The relationship implicit in relaxation can operate on the individual level just as well as on the group level. Group psychology will then have to be taken into consideration.

(c) The Psychotherapeutic Factor

The didactic and physiotherapeutic factors also comprise an important psychotherapeutic element. Psychotherapy *per se*, that is to say, the interpersonal relationships existing between the parturient, her doctor, and her group is what will be considered here. The influence of suggestion comes into play at this stage. It is important to understand what is meant by the word suggestion. It is commonly used in a vague and general way; for many it has a perjorative connotation, and can even imply a breaking down of the personality of the patient by an authoritarian doctor. Here the word will be used in a wide sense, and will be applied

AN EXAMINATION OF THE PROBLEMS

to all emotional relationships of a patient in an interpersonal situation with a therapist and with a group. Amongst other things, a modification of the sensibility to pain can result from this. The relationship which is envisaged here has not always an authoritarian side to it.

The pregnant woman can be the object of different types of psychodynamic processes, all aiming at the diminution, or even the suppression, of anxiety and pain. It has been seen in a preceding chapter that little is known about the physiological and psychological mechanisms of these processes. However, an attempt was made by DONOVAN and LANDISBERG [133], in 33 private patients, to study the value of the interpersonal relationship between the doctor and the patient. They formulated the hypothesis that the diminution of anxiety could be obtained via the transference by means of three mechanisms: (1) the substitution of facts for phantasies, (2) the transformation of a dependent passive attitude to an attitude of active participation, and (3) the anxiety reducing function of group work.*

The French worker R. HELD [225] believes that for a full understanding of verbal analgesia it is necessary to bring in a psychoanalytic viewpoint. He stresses the great importance of the transference in the psychological mechanism of analgesia and the success of the method depends on this. If the transference is good and positive it will allow 'letting go', relaxation, and a carefree attitude. The obstetrician and the other members of his team will play the role of the good or the bad mother, or of the terrible or benevolent father, in the woman's unconscious. The personality of the obstetrician will be constantly implicated and the acceptance or refusal of the method will very closely depend on this.†

---

*It is interesting to note that out of 33 unselected women, two alone were considered by the authors to be normal with minimal neurotic traits. Nevertheless, they believe that this diagnostic classification roughly corresponds 'to a cross-section of the population of the more favoured social and economic group'.

†TSOULADZE and COENCA [541] have considered the matter in Pavlovian terms by saying that the results of the method are linked with the Nervous Types, not only of the woman, but also of the doctor. Throughout, however, the Pavlovian approach does not take into account unconscious motivations behind this intersubjective relationship.

This interreaction takes place not only on the verbal, but also on an infra-verbal, level. The woman has also, through her situation, regressed to a very primitive stage of her emotional life. She will therefore be particularly sensitive to the goodness or the aggressiveness of the accoucheur. Infra-verbal communication can take place 'through a look, the touch of a hand, kindness, or brusqueness in muscular movements, etc.'

Held does not underestimate the dynamic effects of education. Thus he says, 'One can easily imagine that the sessions made in a group setting, whose dynamics themselves are very effective, satisfying infantile curiosities which have been formerly prohibited, can also strongly contribute to the raising of certain inhibitions'.

As to the action of physiotherapy he puts forward the idea that the group or individual exercises allow the woman 'to recognize her body in front of others, not only of not being ashamed of it, but even of loving it'. He insists repeatedly on the importance of the hidden deep personality of the obstetrician, on which will depend the acceptance or the refusal of the method; that is to say, consequently, 'the unrolling of this sublime, existential adventure, of the childbirth'.

All these procedures which we have discussed aim at the suppression or at least the diminution of pain, which has no useful function in childbirth, and may even be harmful. But pain has been given a value from the moral and psychological point of view. In the Bible it is written 'In pain will you bring forth children'. This implies for many Christians that pain is inescapable and has a redemptory value. Recently Pope Pius XII has quite equivocably dissipated these views in approving of the psychological methods of preparation for painless childbirth [3].

In quite another way, psychoanalysts have attempted to attach importance to the pain of childbirth, giving it the useful function of absorbing a certain amount of feminine masochism, and thus allowing the expiation of unconscious guilt.* DEUTSCH [126]

---

*We asked a well-known child analyst if she thought that the pain of childbirth served a useful purpose in women's lives. She replied that, personally, she would have preferred not to suffer, and that this hypothesis was undoubtedly put forward by male analysts. As La Rochefoucault wrote 'we all have plenty of strength to endure the misfortunes of others'.

believes that 'a moderate amount of masochism is normal, and aids in toleration of the pain that women must undergo in the course of reproduction.' Doubtless we must not misunderstand this word 'masochism'. Davidson has said 'It is significant therefore to distinguish between the psychologically destructive expression of neurotic masochism and a healthy exercise of the ability to master pain'. Deutsch finds the method of Read interesting for it shows some advantages over methods of drug anaesthesia by being non-traumatic, and by not depriving the woman of an important emotional experience. Read's method allows the woman, on the contrary, to take an active part in her childbirth and to be in constant contact with the child. Finally she criticizes, on a theoretical level, some of the concepts: the method, she thinks, underestimates interpersonal relationships and unconscious motivations, nor does it take sufficient account of the organic causes of pain.

6. ATTEMPTED FORMULATION

As we have seen, the problem of the psychophysiological mechanisms underlying the analgesia in the different psychological methods (hypnosuggestive, psychoprophylactic and natural childbirth) is a complex one. It may be useful to try to formulate some hypotheses whilst recognizing that these are necessarily tentative and schematic.

The total abolition of pain during childbirth in all women who have been 'prepared' certainly cannot be maintained; but these methods often diminish the pain in various degrees, and sometimes produce a complete absence of pain. How does this happen? In order to simplify the problem it can be considered under two heads: (1) the analgesic effect produced by the action on anxiety, and (2) the direct psychological action on the pain itself quite apart from the question of anxiety.

Under the first heading, it will be recalled that Read insists that there is a relationship between fear and pain in childbirth. Fear encompasses many feelings—conscious and unconscious fear, conscious and unconscious anxiety. The relation between anxiety and pain is complex and little is known concerning it. It is a complex problem of psychodynamic relations in the pregnant woman's personality. Many authors recognize that anxiety produces pain. But one can even conceive that anxiety, at a very deep level, can lead to a painless delivery through a mechanism of denial. Thus one can sometimes see neurotic women have painless deliveries. But in general one admits that the suppression of anxiety can have an analgesic effect. In spite of the difficulty of its experimental verification (in contrast for instance, to the analgesia produced by suggestion) the anxiety-pain concept should be retained as a clinical approach and a fruitful hypothesis for further research.

Under the second heading, psychological analgesia itself operates on the relational level at the level of the intersubjective dimension of the pain.

In the U.S.A., as in the Soviet Union, discussions have been concerned with the pain relieving action of the two methods (the educational, and the hypnosuggestive methods): is it based on the same psychophysiological mechanism, or are two mechanisms at work? Is suggestion the only common factor in all the techniques? Opinions differ among those Anglo-Saxon authors amongst whom the psychological factor is considered pre-eminent, as well as among the Russian authors where a more physiological frame of reference is in use.

For the Russians with their physiological bias, the analgesia in both methods (both the hypnosuggestive and psychoprophylactic methods) results from the action of words on the pregnant or parturient woman.* Some consider the essential factor here is that of suggestion, others that it is of only secondary importance. Velvovski has attempted to differentiate the methods on physiological grounds. The hypnosuggestive method could be formulated as hypnosis-inhibition-therapy, the psychoprophylactic as education-activation-prophylaxis. His views have not been received with favour by the majority of other Russian workers, nor is his thesis supported by sufficient physiological proof. The physiologists themselves maintain that an inhibitory mechanism enters into the production of the analgesia produced by psychological means.

But the concept of this mechanism still requires further exploration.

*The verbal relationship does not embrace the whole problem of interpersonal communication. Speech is certainly of fundamental importance, but other factors occur. AJURIAGURRAE, in his contribution to the Symposium in Paris (1957) entitled 'The integration of pain' said 'An experimenter can produce in his subject a greater or lesser modification of the capacity to suffer. This is not necessarily at the verbal level alone, but is also on the level of the non-verbal emotional relationship' [10]. We would rather speak of 'relational analgesia'.

AN EXAMINATION OF THE PROBLEMS

The electrophysiological objectivation of inhibition accompanying a stimulation in the laboratory animal is only just beginning. So far only very simple stimuli are involved. In man, on the other hand, the emotional significance of the stimulus radically alters the problem.

At the psychological level it is just as difficult to differentiate the essentials of the two methods; the clinical approach might be a useful one. It cannot be denied that suggestion plays a part in all the psychological methods. It is of first importance in the hypnosuggestive method; less so in the others. The analgesia produced by psychological means operates at more than one level; this multiplicity of levels also exists both with regard to motivations and reactions. The early observations in the nineteenth century revealed the diversity of reaction in women submitted to hypnosuggestive procedures (real analgesia, influence on the behaviour, amnesia, etc.). Although the concept of suggestion may not be as yet completely elucidated, it is clear that it works at a relational level. Analgesia produced by suggestion operates within the framework of the doctor-patient relationship. This is also present in the other methods; it is spread over the whole team, its analgesiant effect remains in a somewhat weaker form. But analgesia produced by suggestion is not the only factor in the educational methods. Other levels are concerned—psychodynamic mechanisms are submitted to more complex modifications.*

Schematically, it could be said that 'educational' psychotherapy in the preparation work particularly effect anxiety (which increases or produces the pain), whilst the 'suggestive' relationship† works on the 'organic' pain, independent of the anxiety. In this sense, the action of the educational methods could be considered to be prophylactic, and the hypnosuggestive method as therapeutic.‡ This dissociation is schematic and operational, because anxiety can just as well be suppressed in the 'suggestive' relationship, which is also present in the educational relationship.

The concept of a multiplicity of levels of integration for pain is

---

*This is the difference between suggestive and non-suggestive psychotherapy. It is sometimes difficult to separate these particularly in the case of analgesia.

†A relationship needing further study.

‡Velvovski's 'Therapy-prophylaxis' concept might be interesting, when transposed into psychological terms.

essential in order to understand this latter, just as for the analgesia. Early experiments revealed the multiple reactions possible in the hypnotic methods; in the educational methods it is also relevant, but yet other motivations may also appear. Neurophysiologically this difference of levels is impossible to apprehend in the present state of our knowledge. A clinical approach bearing on reactions and motivations, both conscious and unconscious, before, during and after childbirth would shed some light on the problem at the psychological level. For instance, is there a correlation between the kind of motivation and the kind of reaction which occurs? The present state of research does not allow an answer to the question. The establishment of correlations between neurophysiological and psychological data is the task of the future.

7. THE PARTICIPATION OF THE HUSBAND

The importance of the husband's participation in psychosomatic methods is stressed by many writers. It was first estimated in relation to the success of the method. Some writers assigned a particularly important role to the husband's participation, even explaining the failures by its absence (HERNANDEZ JIMENEZ [228]). A special course for husbands has been begun by French practitioners (BOURREL et al. [58]).

It has also been claimed that the husband's participation 'diminishes the emotional transference of the woman to her obstetrician' and enables the latter 'to put at once a share of the responsibility on the husband's shoulders and to make him aware of his role in the process of childbirth' (LAMAZE and VELAY [305]).*

Other writers go further, and see in the collaboration of the husband and wife during pregnancy and childbirth, a factor which helps to make for better emotional equilibrium between the couple (Read, Thoms, Laird and Hogan).

The husband's participation can be considered from two points of view: his collaboration in the preparation and his presence during the childbirth itself. The first offers no difficulties. No one is opposed to the husband taking part in the preparation (training

*Perhaps in some cases the doctor protects himself against this emotional transference and thus its diminution will be useful to him, at the same time as to the woman. All this confirms the importance of the doctor's personality (or of his Nervous Type) in the use of the method.

in the exercises, etc.). But there is not the same agreement concerning his presence during the childbirth. For instance, the Russians completely oppose this, as is shown by their criticisms of Dobbin's article [582].

Some German workers are of the same opinion. HELLMANN [227], for instance, believes that however strong the man may be he cannot always endure the sight of his wife's suffering, or of accidents arising during the course of childbirth (such as haemorrhages). He very much doubts whether the woman's natural modesty would not be upset by the presence of her husband, and adds that his collaboration can increase the feeling of camaraderie between the couple but can also diminish the sexual desire of the husband.

Other writers attach much importance, sometimes even a capital importance, to the presence of the husband in the labour ward. 'You will live her childbirth over with her'* M. and A. Bourrel and Jeanson say to their patients' husbands, 'With her you will also hear the first cry of your child'.

THOMS and WIEDENBACH [535] and VOLLMER [569] use the husband to carry out back-rubbing. He can also be taught how to time the contractions and how to train his wife in the exercises (MURPHY [377]). At the period of dilatation he can also distract his wife by playing cards with her, or by listening to the radio (LAIRD and HOGAN [292]).

RANSOM [450] recommends the presence of the husband if the wife wants it. This creates a feeling of confidence. It also produces, according to Lamaze and Vellay, a motivation for the success of the method; the woman wants to show her husband that she can

---

*This idea brings up the custom of 'couvade'—'a custom in which the husband takes his wife's place in the bed—is taken care of in her stead, and plays this part for a variable time'. (VAN GENNEP [547]). Couvade has been practised by many peoples and has been verified in the Basque Country, in France at the end of the nineteenth century. Perhaps there is a certain deep correspondence of a sociopsychological nature between this custom and the presence of the husband in the psychosomatic methods. In any case this might be a problem for future research. In primitive peoples the husband sometimes attends the delivery. JOCHELSON [252] reports that in Yakoughirs, the husband and sometimes the father of the parturient woman are present at the childbirth, and take an active part in applying pressure to the woman's belly.

go through childbirth without feeling pain. Laird and Hogan believe, however, that some women prefer to remain with the obstetrician or the nurse, whilst their husband stays at home. Some husbands prefer to be in the labour ward—others not. The staff—the members of the team—sometimes complain of the husband's agitation—in other cases his presence has a happy effect.

VOLLMER [569] believes that it is sometimes desirable for the husbands to assist in the birth, but not always so. He has noticed that women who might have shown anxiety on account of the absence of their husband were reassured by his arrival.

ECONOMIDES and VERMOREL [143] feel that it is a mistake to allow the husband to help his wife alone without the presence of a competent person.

AUZIAS [27], a psychologist in Paris, is very much in favour of the presence of the husband, who in certain cases of difficult childbirth is the one person who can most easily obtain the maximum efforts from his wife to control herself. In her own experience, the proportion of husbands who are too emotional to help at all in the childbirth is no more than two or three per cent. She carried out a study on 70 women who had been treated by Drs. Vellay and Randon. She collected the experiences of the women themselves, their husbands, the obstetricians, midwives and teachers. Eighty-three per cent of the husbands were present at the labours and their presence was helpful in 94 per cent of cases. It gives their wives proof of their affection and of the absence of danger. For the husbands it was, as one of them has said, 'a human experience both passionate and enriching'.

In conclusion we feel that it is difficult to give general directives with regard to the presence of the husband. Different views will be held in each different country, according to their customs and habits, and its use depends on the personalities of the obstetrician and the midwife, as well as of the husband and wife.

8. THE RESULTS

The results can be considered in several ways.

(a) *Analgesia and Behaviour*

The primary aim of the methods is to produce an analgesia. This has been attained in varying degrees, but, on the whole, experience has shown that the methods offer other advantages such as a disciplining effect on the behaviour of the parturient, obstetrical and medical advantages in general, and, finally, social and psychological advantages. As most authors have stressed, the chief difficulty in the evaluation of analgesia, is due to the absence of criteria by which pain can be measured. The subjective character of the woman's statements and of the observer's conclusions cannot be overlooked.

This question has been particularly studied by FREEDMAN, REDLICH and their colleagues [147, 148]. They found that mothers tended to believe that they had suffered less and co-operated more than they actually had, at least in the observer's opinion. In all cases, the observation of the resident physician and the nurse presented a higher degree of correlation with each other than with the mother. The writers found no prominent amnesic features in the patients, but partial or slight amnesias were present which might have distorted their opinions. This leads to the problem of the relationship between amnesia and analgesia, so remarked on by the other writers, and so difficult to resolve. Simply, it can be said that both processes are in part motivated by existing emotional factors.

In the clinical observations of the older writers it is clear that the attitude of the women towards pain can take different forms. For instance, a calm behaviour does not mean that there is no pain. The new Soviet outlook, which considers the results of the Psychoprophylactic Method from two aspects, those of the analgesia and of behaviour, takes better account of these facts. According to the most recent Russian statistics, the positive results relating to behaviour are twice as good as on those relating directly to the analgesia itself.

These two types of result spring from the interpersonal relationship existing at all stages of the preparation, and whose modes of action are of both a rational and irrational character. *It can be said that the achievements of behaviour obtained by learning, although unconscious motivations are always of importance, are largely the result of conscious, voluntary, and active factors. The analgesia itself would be the result of irrational affective factors, which enter into what is called suggestion (hypnotic analgesia, for instance, is an extreme example of this), or any other type of psychotherapy.*

Doubtless these two kinds of results are not acquired in an independent manner, and there is a constant interaction between them. For instance, disciplined behaviour, itself of great importance, can have an analgesic effect, if only through the possibilities which it offers to the pregnant woman of carrying out the pain reducing exercises.

(b) Medical and Obstetrical Advantages

These will not be discussed in detail. They have been recognized by most authors. Briefly listing some of them, there is a favourable influence on the pathology of pregnancy, a diminution of the length of labour, a diminution in the complications during the course of childbirth, a reduction in obstetrical interventions, a favourable action on the puerperal period, a diminution in neonatal mortality and in the number of resuscitations of the newborn child which are needed, as well as in a lesser frequency of anoxemic encephalopathies with later complications.

(c) Mental Hygiene

Pregnancy and childbirth pose numerous problems of mental hygiene, constituting, as they do, primordial affective experiences for the woman, and also as a result of the effects which they can have on the child. These problems may surpass in importance those of the analgesia, and the medical and obstetrical benefits so closely linked with that analgesia. Unfortunately, the matter can only be briefly discussed here.

The mental health of the woman will have repercussions on the course of pregnancy (vomiting, abortions, etc.), the quality of the labour, the analgesia at the time of the delivery and the behaviour of the parturient. But her mental hygiene has a wider significance, especially with regard to the mother–child relationship. It is only over the last 15 years or so that this relationship has been studied, and in the United States a reawakening of interest has been stimulated by the considerable increase in mental disorder over the last 50 years. Psychoanalysis had in fact drawn attention to the importance of the early years of life in emotional development, and in the disturbances of emotion which can so influence the whole of a person's life. The problem of good or bad 'mothering' has thus been raised, as well as problems of rooming-in, of breast-feeding and of natural childbirth. The latter, in fact, allows the woman to live through the experience of childbirth, which is the beginning of the mother-child relationships apart from the relationships during pregnancy. During the pregnancy itself a good preparation, carried out with the help of psychologists, and oriented towards the psychological problems of the woman, can already in this prenatal stage exert an influence on those relationships.

In 1947 to 1948 two conferences were organized by the Macy Foundation and were devoted to the problem of early infancy. MOLONEY [371] reported that between 1880 and 1943 the proportion of patients in psychiatric hospitals in America increased from 80 to 365 per 100,000. He stated that during the Second World War 51 per cent of rural recruits and 41 per cent of urban recruits needed treatment for psychiatric disorder. On the other hand in Okinawa, there were less than 250 mental patients amongst 350,000 inhabitants. There, 'mothering' is particularly good, for instance the mothers are never separated from their children, which they breast-feed.

Even though the first relationships between the child and the mother are very important for its future emotional development, they do not alone furnish an explanation for the origin of mental disorder. Statistical proof is still lacking to link mental disturbance to breast-feeding, or to the precocious separation of the child from the mother. It is clear, however, that events such as the experience of childbirth, breast-feeding, and rooming-in, discerningly carried out, can have only a happy influence on the relationships between the mother and the child.

Finally, the emotional problems linked with pregnancy and childbirth which may influence marital relationships, should be briefly mentioned.

In the American literature some systematic studies have been made on the mental hygiene of mothers-to-be, quite independent of any method of psychosomatic preparation. The introduction of these methods, however, offers the greatest possibilities of contact with the future mothers, and on this account opens up a vast field of research, and of psychological work. The problems of psychoprophylaxis and psychotherapy confront us at all stages of preparation and childbirth. The interpersonal relationships occur at several levels: between the woman, the medical and nursing staff, and the group. Needless to say, the mental health of the medical and nursing services is also of great importance.*

*KUBIE [289] writes concerning this: ' "Educated childbirth" means educating not only the woman but also the young house officer. . . . We often forget that some young doctors hate obstetrics, women and babies. Moreover, some of those who go into obstetrics have this as their unconscious bias, just as some people who hate books become librarians or publishers.'

CONCLUSION

Throughout history men have sought to diminish, or even to suppress, the pain of childbirth, at first by magical means, later by more scientific methods. In the nineteenth century modern medicine introduced anaesthesia and analgesia produced by chemical substances. These pharmacological methods were not free from toxicity for both mother and child, and moreover suppressed an important emotional experience in the woman's life. Other methods were therefore sought for. Psychologically produced analgesia was demonstrated experimentally, about the beginning of the nineteenth century, using hypnosis. Childbirth without pain was carried out under hypnosis, but only on a small scale. Hypnosis was shown to have a particular psychotherapeutic effect, but it always aroused prejudice, and does so even today, in spite of the caution shown by men such as Charcot, Bernheim, Freud, Pavlov, Forel and others who used it. In these circumstances new methods were developed, which did not directly rely on hypnosuggestive techniques. The first was that of Read, the second is the work of the Russian psychiatrist Velvovski, and his team. The two methods, the differences between which are minimal in practice, are based on didactic, physiotherapeutic and psychotherapeutic elements. Read began his work as a result of his fruitful intuition, the researches of Velvovski followed on his experiences of hypnosuggestive analgesia in obstetrics, which had already convinced him of the reality of verbal analgesia. The two methods are both effective; their theoretical bases are unclear and controversial. Without minimizing the role of didactic and physiotherapeutic factors, the psychotherapeutic factor is of most importance in the production of the analgesia, and is at work at all the stages of the method. It must be stressed that psychotherapy is here being used on healthy persons. Psychotherapy brings with it a comprehensive and human attitude towards the mothers-to-be. The psychological and physiological mechanisms of the analgesia produced by psychological means in the framework of an interpersonal relationship, are still obscure. The results of the analgesia are difficult to evaluate in the absence of objective criteria of pain. In addition to the analgesia the methods have other positive results, both medical, and obstetrical. They have brought about an important advance in the mental hygiene of the mother and of the nursling by dignifying woman's status and humanizing the act of childbirth. These diverse results are in line with the concepts of modern psychosomatic medicine, which stress the importance of emotional factors in biological phenomena. The introduction of psychosomatic methods to obstetrics marks a considerable medical and psychosocial advance.

BIBLIOGRAPHY

1. P. ABOULKER and L. CHERTOK, Étude psychosomatique de la cystalgie à urines claires. *Presse Médicale* (1952) 60, No. 68, 1448–1450.
2. M. ABRAMSON and W. T. HERON, Objective evaluation of hypnosis in obstetrics; preliminary report. *Amer. J. Obstet. Gynec.* (1950). **59**, 1069–1074.
3. Painless childbirth, Discourse delivered by Pius XII before the International Assembly of Gynaecologists and Obstetricians at Rome, January 1956. *Osservatore Romano*, 9–10 January (1956).
4. L'accouchement sans douleur à Genève. *Méd. et. Hyg.*, Genève, (1955) **13**, 176.
5. L'accouchement sans douleur. *ELLE encyclopedie, Librairie Arthème Fayard* (1957). Préface de P. Vellay.
6. E. C. AIRAPETIANZ, Concerning signalization arising in the genital region. *Probl. Kortiko-Vistzeralnoi Patolog.*, Academy of Medical Sciences, Moscow (1949) 73–92.
7. E. C. AIRAPETIANZ, Researches into the mechanism of the internal analyses of higher nervous activity. *Communication to the XIX International Congress of Physiology.* Montreal (1953).
8. J. DE AJURIAGUERRA and J. GARCIA BADARACCO, Les thérapeutiques de relaxation en médecine psychosomatique. *Pr. Méd.* (1953) **61**, 316–320.
9. J. DE AJURIAGUERRA, J. GARCIA BADARACCO, E. TRILLAT and G. SOUBIRAN, Traitement de la crampe des écrivains par la relaxation. (Le processus de guérison à partir de l'expérience tonique). *Encéphale* (1956) **45**, 141–171.
10. J. DE AJURIAGUERRA, L'intégration de la douleur. *La Journée d'Études sur les Méthodes psychologiques en Analgésie Obstétricale*, Paris, 7 April (1957).
11. Th. ALAJOUANINE et al. *La Douleur et les Douleurs.* Masson & Co. Paris (1957).
12. F. ALEXANDER, *Psychosomatic Medicine.* Allen & Unwin (1952).
13. G. AMBROSE and G. NEWBOLD, *A Handbook of Medical Hypnosis.* Baillière, Tindall and Cox, London (1956).
14. C. P. AMFITEATROV, Hypnotic obstetrical analgesia. *Akush. Ginek.* (1937), No. 12, 17–23.
15. R. ANGELERGUES, Quelques critiques sur les conceptions théoriques et la pratique de Read dans l'accouchement sans douleur. *Bull. Cerc Claude Bernard* (1954) No. 8, 6–7.
16. R. ANGELERGUES, La conception pavlovienne de la douleur dans l'accouchement. *Rev. Nouvelle Méd.* (1954) **1**, No. 3, 9–32.
17. R. ANGELERGUES, E. BAULIEU, V. LAFITTE, J. LEVY and R. ROELENS, Pavlov et Pavlovisme. *Edit. les Essais de la NC;* Paris (1957).

18. R. ANGELERGUES, Naissance et disparition de la douleur. *Pensée* (1955) No. 60, 43–65.
19. P. K. ANOKHINE, On the physiological mechanisms of pain reactions. *Kiev Congress* (90), 70–80.
20. A. M. ARNOLDOVA, The influence of psychoprophylactic preparation on the course of childbirth particularly in the first phase. *Akouch. i. Guin.*, 6 (1957) 30–33.
21. E. ARON, *Histoire de l'Anesthésie*. Expansion Scientifique Française, Paris (1954).
22. I. B. ASSATUROV, M. T. LEBED, V. M. KANIEVSKAIA and N. A. BACHNINSKAIA, The psychoprophylactic method of analgesia. *Akush. Ginek.* (1955) No. 1, 36–39.
23. S. N. ASTAKHOV and N. I. BESKROVNAIA, An experience of painless childbirth using the method of verbal activity, in pregnant women and in the parturient. *Leningrad Congress* (89), 48–54.
24. AUARD MARTINEZ DIAZ, Quelques faits d'anesthésie chirurgicale sous l'influence de la suggestion. *Rev. Hypnot., Paris* (1892), 309–313.
25. A. AUVARD and SECHEYRON, L'hypnotisme et la suggestion en obstétrique. *Archives de Tocologie* (1888), 26–40, 78–104, 146–176.
26. A. AUVARD and VARNIER, Accouchement chez une hypnotique. *Ann. Gynéc. Obstet.* (1887), 363.
27. G. AUZIAS, Personal communication.
28. J. BABINSKI, De l'hypnose en thérapeutique et en médecine légale. *Semaine Médicale, Paris* (1910).
29. E. BANSILLON and A. NOTTER, Accouchement sans douleur ou accouchement sans crainte. *Lyon. Méd.* (1954) **86**, 433–446.
30. E. BANSILLON and A. NOTTER, L'influence de la relaxation contrôlée durant la grossesse sur la marche de l'accouchement (81 observations de tuberculeuses enceintes ayant subi la cure sanatoriale). *Bull. Féd. Soc. Gyn. Obst. franç.* (1954) **6**, 212–213.
31. H. DE BARAHONA FERNANDEZ, O falso dontrinao na pragmatica medica. *Medico* (1955), No. 213.
32. R. BAUX, Cent premiers cas d'analgésie obstétricale par la méthode psychoprophylactique. *Bull. Féd. Soc. Gyn. Obst. franç.* (1954) **6**, 332–336.
33. R. BAUX and Y. FERRIER, Notre expérience de l'analgésie obstétricale par psychoprophylaxie en clientèle privée (700 cas). *Bull. Féd. Soc. Gyn. Obst. franç.*, (1955) **7**, 587–591.
34. H. BEAUNIS, *Le Somnambulisme Provoqué: Études Physiologiques et Psychologiques*. Baillère et Fils, Paris (1887).
35. W. M. BECHTEREW, *La Suggestion et son Rôle dans la Vie Sociale*, Boulangé, Paris (1910).
36. P. A. BELOCHAPKO, *Leningrad Congress* (89) p. 67.
37. P. A. BELOCHAPKO, The practice of psychoprophylactic preparation for childbirth in the obstetrical and gynaecological institutions of the Academy of Medical Sciences of the USSR. *Kiev Congress* (90) 34–38.

38. P. A. BELOCHAPKO and A. M. FOI, *Analgesia and the Acceleration of Labour*. Medquiz, Moscow (1954).
39. U. BERGANDER, Einige Erfahrungen mit psychoprophylactischen Entbindungen. *Z. ärzt. Fortbild.* (1956) **24**, 1013–1019.
40. S. BERLIOZ, L'accouchement sans douleur dans un Hôpital de district. *Rev. Méd. Suisse.* (1956) **76**, 878–882.
41. C. BERMUDES, Bases cientificas do parto sem dor. *J. Med. Pharm. Port.* (1955) **28**, 797–801.
42. H. BERNHEIM. *De la Suggestion et de ses Applications à la Thérapeutique.* O. Doin, Paris (1891). 3rd ed.
43. H. BERNHEIM, *Jubilé*, 12 November (1910).
44. N. I. BESKROVNAIA, Clinical details of the course of complicated deliveries in women prepared by the psychoprophylactic method., *Akush. Ginek.* (1955) No. 4, 7–11.
45. R. BLANCHARD, Un nouveau procédé d'anesthésie. *Progr. méd. Paris* (1881) **9**, 141–142.
46. E. BLEULER, Zur Psychologie der hypnose. *Münch. med. Wschr.* (1889) No. 5, 76–77.
47. J. R. BLOOS, Cause of fear among obstetric patients. *J. Amer. Med. Ass.* (1950) **144**, 1358–1361.
48. A. BOCCI, G. CHIAUDANO, L. DAVITTI, G. PINOLI and I. TERZI, *Il Parto Naturale con il Metodo Psico-fisioterapico: Fondamenti Téorici e Risultato Clinico.* Minerva Medica, Turin (1956).
49. A. BOCCI, G. CHIAUDANO, L. DAVITTI, G. PINOLI and I. TERZI, *La Preparazione Psicofisica al Parto.* Minerva Medica, Turin (1956).
50. A. BOCCI and L. DAVITTI, Le déclenchement du travail en dehors de l'époque prévue et ses répercussions psychiques chez la gestante soumise à la préparation psychophysique. *La Journée d'Études sur les Méthodes Psychologiques en Analgésie Obstétricale*, Paris, 7 April (1957).
51. V. G. BOJOVSKI and I. I. TOUREVSKI, Hypnosis during Childbirth. *Kazansk. med. Zh.* (1927), 226–230.
52. BONNE, Über Suggestion und Hypnose in der Praxis. *Dtsch. med. Wschr.* (1919), 132–133.
53. M. BONVALLET, Donnée neurophysiologiques récentes concernant l'organisation centrale du système nerveux et le rôle de la formation réticulée du tronc cérébral. *Récent Progrès en Physiologie*, Presses Universitaires de France, Paris (1956), 1–12.
54. W. G. A. BONWILL, Rapid breathing a pain-obtunder in minor surgery, obstetrics, the general practice of medicine and of dentistry. *Philadelphia Medical Times*, Philadelphia (1880) **10**, 1879–1880.
55. I. A. BOTKINE. *Hypnotism on Gynaecology and Obstetrics.* Moscow (1897).
56. BOULAVINTSEVA, Quoted by TEREKHOVA [523].
57. A. BOURREL, Les cours préparatoires. *Revue de la Nouvelle Médecine* (1954) No. 3, 33–61.

58. M. Bourrel, A. Bourrel and C. Jeanson, *La Méthode Complète de Préparation a l'Accouchement sans Douleur*. Seuil, Paris (1957).
59. J. Braid, *Neurypnology*. J. Churchill, London (1843).
60. M. Brenman, Perception of pain and some factors that modify it. *Problems of Consciousness* (405), 103–122.
61. M. Brenman, M. Gill and R. P. Knight, Spontaneous fluctuations in depth of hypnosis and their implications for ego-function. *Int. Psycho-Anal.* (1952) 22–33.
62. P. Broca, Note sur une nouvelle méthode anesthésique. *C.R. Acad. Sci., Paris* (1859) **49**, 902–905.
63. P. Broca, Sur l'anesthésie chirurgicale provoquée par l'hypnotisme. *Bull. Soc. Chir. Paris* (1859), Librairie de Victor Masson, Paris (1806), 247–271.
64. W. L. Von Brunn, Die Anfange der Hypnotischen Anaesthesie. *Dtsch. med. Wschr.* (1954), 336–340.
65. A. S. Burger, La relaxation, la psychothérapie et le problème des nevroses dans l'oeuvre de J. H. Schultz. *Evolution Psychiatrique* (1957) 163–173.
66. A. J. Burger, Psychothérapie de relaxation. *Encyclopédie médico-chirurgicale Volume de Psychiatrie* (1957).
67. Burger-Eastman, Die werdende Mutter. Mueller-Verlag (1949).
68. C. W. F. Burnett, The value of antenatal exercises. *J. Obstet. Gynaec., Brit. Emp.* (1956) **63**, 40–57.
69. R. Burthiault and C. Garnier, En marge de la préparation à l'accouchement dit sans douleur; les douleurs de reins au cours de la grossesse et pendant le travail. *Gynéc. et Obstét.* (1956) **55**, 83–86.
70. C. Lee Buxton, Prepared childbirth and rooming-in at Yale. *Penn. med. J.* (1957) **60**, 171–176.
71. K. M. Bykov, *The Cerebral Cortex and Internal Organs*. 3rd ed. Gos. izd. Med. Lit., Moscow (1954). French transl. Moscow (1956).
72. K. M. Bykov, New ideas on the physiology and the pathology of the cortex. 19*th Int. Congr. Physiology, Montreal* (1953).
73. K. M. Bykov, Physiology and psychosomatic problems. *Probl. Kortiko-Vistzeralnoi Patolog.* Academy of Medical Sciences, Moscow (1949) 5–18.
74. J. Cech, Psychoprophylactic preparation in pathological pregnancies. *Prakt. Lek.*, Praha (1953) **33**, 118–120.
75. J. Chaigneau, *Étude Comparative des Différents États Anesthésiques Employés dans les Accouchements Naturels*. G. Steinheil, Paris (1890).
76. G. Chapus, Quelques réflexions sur l'accouchement psychoprophylactique. *Bull. Féd. Soc. Gyn. Obst. franç.* (1955) **7**, 170–172.
77. J. Charcot, Leçon sur catalepsie et le somnambulisme provoqués (Communication by P. Richer). *Progr. med., Paris* (1878) 973–975.
78. J. Charcot, Complete works in nine volumes.
79. J. Charcot, Leçons du Mardi à la Salpêtrière. Policlinique (1887–

1888). Vol. 1. *Progr. méd.* 2nd ed., Louis Bataille, Paris (1892). Vol. 2. *Progr. méd.*, E. Lecronier and Babé, Paris (1889).
80. L. CHERTOK, Hypnose et suggestion. *Encyclopédie médico-chirurgicale. Psychiatrie* 37, 810 E. 10, Paris (1955).
81. L. CHERTOK, Utilisation médicale de l'hypnose. A propos du récent rapport de la British Medical Association (431). *Gaz. Méd. Fr.* (1955) **62**, 853–854.
82. L. CHERTOK, Étude de la psychoprophylaxie des douleurs de l'accouchement. *Sem. Hôp. Paris* (1956) **32**, 2619–2626.
83. L. CHERTOK, P. ABOULKER and M. CAHEN, Perspective psychosomatique en urologie. *Evolut. psychiat.* (1953) **3**, 457–473.
84. L. CHERTOK and M. CAHEN, Facteurs transférentiels en hypnose. *Acta Psychother., Psychosom. Orthopaed., Bâle.* (1955) Suppl., **3**, 334–342.
85. L. CHERTOK and P. KRAMARZ, Hypnose et EEG. *Sem. Hôp. Paris* (1955) **31**, RM136–RM143.
86. L. CHERTOK, Evolution des idées sur l'analgésie psychologique en obstétrique. *La Journée d'Études sur les Méthodes Pyschologiques en Analgésie Obstétricale*, Paris, 7 April (1957).
87. L. CHERTOK, L' 'Accouchement naturel' et l' 'Accouchement psychoprophylactique', *Concours méd.* (1957) No. 47, 5105–5107.
88. CHESTOPAL, See PLATONOV and CHESTOPAL [429].
89. G. CHIAUDANO and G. PINOLI, Eléments d'une méthodologie moderne audio-visuelle dans le conditionnement de la gestante. *La Journée d'Études sur les Méthodes Psychologiques en Analgésie Obstétricale*, Paris, 7 April (1957).
90. V. N. CHICHKOVA, R. M. BRONSTEIN, E. I. IVANOV and P. NIKOULINE, *Psychoprophylactic obstétrical analgesie*. Leningrad Congress **76**, 54–59.
91. V. N. CHICHKOVA and I. P. IVANOV, Psychoprophylactic preparation in pathological pregnancies. *Akush. Ginek.* (1955) No. 4, 12–17.
92. R. IA. CHLIFER, Verbal analgesia in childbirth. *Psychotherapia, Kharkov* (1930), 307–318.
93. E. A. CHOUGOM [558] Lectures 13, 14 and 15.
94. P. L. CHOUPIK, The present state of psychoprophylactic preparation for labour, and tasks for a larger application of this method in Obstetrical Institutions in the U.S.S.R. *Kiev Congress*, (90), 3–11.
95. R. N. CLARK, Training method for childbirth utilizing hypnosis. *Amer. J. of Obstet. Gynec.* (1956) **72**, 1302–1304.
96. J. CLOQUET, Ablation d'un cancer du sein pendant le sommeil magnétique. *Arch. gen. Méd.* (1829) **20**, 131.
97. J. COENCA, *La Psychoprophylaxie de la Douleur dans l'Accouchement.* Thesis, Paris (1954).
98. Colloquium on 'L'activité électrique du cerveau en relation avec les phénomènes psychologiques', 7–12 November (1955) at Marseilles. *Conditionnement, Comportement et Réactivité en Electroencéphalographie.* Masson and Co., Paris (1957).

99. Congress on obstetrical analgesia, 29–31 January (1951) at Leningrad. *Obezbolivanie v rodakh (Obstetrical Analgesia)* A. P. NICOLAIEV, Academy of Medical Sciences, Moscow (1952). Translated into German as *Schmerzausschaltung*, Geburt, Vebverlag Volk and Gesundheit, Berlin (1953).
100. Congress on the advancement of the psychoprophylactic preparation for labour. 10–14 February (1956) at Kiev. *Akush. Ginek.* (1956).
101. 17th Congress of the German Gynaecological Society (Verhandlungen der Deutschen Geselschaft für (Gynaekologie), Innsbruck, 10–22 June (1922). *Arch. Gynaek.* (1922) 117.
102. C. E. COOKE and A. E. VAN VOGT, *The Hypnotism Handbook.* Griffin Publishing Company, Los Angeles, U.S.A. (1956).
103. H. CORBIN, Meeting the needs of mothers and babies. *Amer. J. Nurs.* (1957) **57**.
104. A. COTA-GUERRA, Fisiopatologia cortico-visceral e o parto sem dor. *O Médico* (1955) **6**, No. 226.
105. P. COTTEEL, S. COTTEEL and L. CACAN, L'accouchement sans douleur par la méthode psychoprophylactique. Nos résultats de 18 mois. *Lille médical*, (1956) **1**, 181–186.
106. J. COURTOIS, Accouchement sans crainte, accouchement sans douleur, accouchement normal. *Rev. Hyg. et Méd. Soc.*, Paris (1956), **4**, 480–488.
107. W. A. CRAMOND, Psychological aspects of uterine dysfunction. *Lancet*, (1954) ii, 1241–1245.
108. Dr. CUTTER, Traitements magnétiques. Accouchement. *J. Magnét.* (1845) 115–116.
109. E. DABROWSKI, Résultats de ia psychoprophylaxie des douleurs de l'accouchement. *Pol. med. Wkly* **11**, 1786–1790.
110. V. I. DANILEVSKI, List of Danilevski's works in Finkelstein's Monograph: *Vassilii Jakovlevitch, Danilevski.* Acad. Sciences, U.S.S.R. (1955).
111. J. LE DANTEC, *A Propos de l'Accouchement sans Douleur.* Thesis, Paris (1956).
112. S. N. DAVIDENKOV, *Leningrad Congress* (89) 71.
113. H. B. DAVIDSON, Education for childbirth. *N.Y. Med.* (1952) **8**.
114. H. B. DAVIDSON, The psychosomatic aspects of educated childbirth. *N.Y. St. J. Med.* (1953) **53**, 2499–2510.
115. G. DEAVER, Clinical aspects and cerebral palsy. *J. Phys. Ment. Rehabilitation* (1950).
116. J. DECHAUME, Psychothérapie et psychophylaxie. *J. Med. Lyon* (1955) **36**, 441–450.
117. J. DEJERINE and E. GAUCKLER, *Les Manifestations Fonctionelles des Psychonévroses.* (1911) Masson and Co., Paris.
118. J. DELAY, *La Psychophysiologie Humaine. Que Sais-je?* Press Univ. de France, Paris (1954).
119. S. T. DE LEE, Hypnotism in pregnancy and labor. *J. Amer. med. Ass.* (1955) **159**, 750–754.

120. S. T. DE LEE and J. I. DUNCAN, Training for natural childbirth. *Amer. J. Nurs.* (1956) **56**, 48–50.
121. J. DE LEEUWE, Psychoprophylaxe ter Opheffing van Barenspyn. *Geneeskundige Bladen uit Kliniek en Laboratorium, Haarlem* (1955), 193–239.
122. P. DELI. and M. BONVALLET, Données expérimentales récentes sur la physiologie du sommeil. G. NORA and M. SAPIR, *Cure de Sommeil.* Masson and Co., Paris (1954), 23–26.
123. G. DELLEPIANE, Il parto senza paura. *Minerva Ginecologica* (1952) **4**, 41–43.
124. G. DELLEPIANE, La preparazione psicofisica al parto ovvero: il parto senza paura. *Minerva Ginecologica,* (1955) **7**, 636–639.
125. M. DEMANGEAT, Les thérapeutiques de relaxation. *Gaz. méd. Fr.* (1956) 1317–1325.
126. H. DEUTSCH, *Psychology of Women. A Psychoanalytic Interpretation.* 2 Vols. (1946) Heinemann.
127. J. H. DIETLIN, *De l'Accouchement Psychoprophylactique.* Thesis, Bordeaux, 29 November (1954) 237.
128. A. C. DOBBIN, Natural childbirth. (Experience of an Australian doctor). *Akush. Ginek.* (1957) **2**, 41–44.
129. M. DOBROVOLSKY, Huit observations d'accouchement sans douleurs sous l'influence de l'hypnotisme. *Rev. Hypnot., Paris.* (1891), 274–277; 310–312.
130. I. DOGANOV, Our results of the use of the psychoprophylactic method in painless childbirth. *Khirurgiia, Sofia,* (1956) **6**, 475–483.
131. A. O. DOLINE and G. M. SALGANNIK, The physiological bases of psychoprophylactic preparation for labour. *Kiev Congress* (90), 47–62.
132. M. I. DONIGUEVITCH, *Psychoprophylaxis of the Pains of Childbirth.* Gosmedizdat, Kiev (1955).
133. P. DONOVAN and S. LANDISBERG, Some psychologic observations of educated childbirth. (104). *N.Y. St. J. Med.* (1953) **6**, 2504–2510.
134. J. DOS SANTOS, Parto sem dor e psicoterapia. *Cadern. cient.* (1956 **4**, No. 3.
135. H. DRAPS and R. SCHOYSMAN, 1000 accouchements 'sans douleur', succes et echecs de la methode psychoprophylactique. *Gyn. et Obst.* (1957) **9**.
136. Dr. DUBOIS, *Les Psychonévroses et leur Traitement Moral.* Masson and Co. (1909), 3rd ed.
137. D. DUMONTPALLIER, De l'analgésie hypnotique dans le travail de l'accouchement. *Rev. Hypnot., Paris* (1887), 258–261.
138. D. DUMONTPALLIER, De l'action de la suggestion pendant le travail de l'accouchement. *Rev. Hypnot., Paris* (1892), 175–177.
139. F. DUNBAR, *Emotions and Bodily Changes. A Survey of Literature on Psychosomatic Interrelationships* 1910–1945. Columbia Univ. Press, New York (1947), 3rd ed.

140. Du Potet, *Traité Complet de Magnétisme Animal.* Félix Alcan, Paris (1904), 6th ed.
141. M. Ebner, Physiotherapy and antenatal care. II. Training for natural childbirth; physical preparation, *Physiotherapy, Lond.* (1955) **41,** 137–142.
142. A. Economides, État actuel de la pratique de l'accouchement sans douleur en France. *Revue de la Nouvelle Médecine,* (1956) **6,** 71–79.
143. A. Economides and H. Vermorel, Quelques considérations théoriques et pratiques sur la méthode psychoprophylactique après une expérience de 400 préparations. *La Journée d'Études sur les Méthodes Psychologiques en Analgésie Obstétricale, Paris,* 7 April (1957).
144. B. Edwards, Quelques faits de suggestion. *Progr. méd. Paris* (1890) 1, 500–502.
145. I. S. Eligulachvili, *Gestation and parturition in the monkey.* Medguiz, Moscow (1956).
146. J. Elliotson, *Numerous Cases of Surgical Operations without Pain in the Mesmeric State,* London, 1843.
147. J. Elliotson, Operations without pain in the mesmeric state. *Zoist,* 1845–1846, 380–389.
148. L. W. Van Eps, Psychoprophylaxis in labour. *Lancet* (1955) ii, 112–115.
149. L. W. Van Eps, De voorbereiding tot de normale bevalling. *Geneesk. Gids* (1955) **33,** 369–367.
150. M. N. Erofeeva, *Electrical Stimulation of the Skin of a Dog as a Conditioned Stimulus for Salivary Activity.* Thesis presented to the Academy of Military Medicine 1912. Reissued in Academy of Medical Sciences of the U.S.S.R. Moscow (1953).
151. J. Esdaile, *Mesmerism in India,* Ed. Esdaile. London (1846).
152. J. Esdaile, *Natural and Mesmeric Clairvoyance with the Practical Application of Mesmerism in Surgery and Medicine.* London, (1852).
153. R. Falk, Ein weiterer Beitrag zur Hypnose in der Geburtshilfe und Gynaekologie. *Zbl. Gynak.* (1922) **17,** 658–661.
154. M. Fanton, De l'accouchement sans souffrance. (Communication given at the Congrès de l'Association Française pour l'Avancement des Sciences). *Arch. Tocologie* (1890), 104–108.
155. M. Fanton, Un accouchement sans douleur sous l'influence de l'hypnotisme. *Rev. Hypnot., Paris* (1891) 150–155.
156. L'Abbé Faria, *De la Cause du Sommeil Lucide ou Étude sur la Nature de l'Homme.* Horiac, Paris (1819); M. Jouve, (1906), 2nd ed.
157. R. Favarel, Le médecin rural devant l'accouchement sans douleur. *Concours Méd.* (1955) **77,** 3233–3239.
158. Fere and Budin, Hypnotisme pendant la grossesse, impossible pendant le travail. Leonard, [320] (1886/87).
159. S. Ferenczi, Introjection and transference, 35–93. (298), Transl. E. Jones; *Jb. Psychoanal.* (1909) **1,** 481. Hogarth Press (1952).

160. A. Gomez Ferreira, Los metodos psicofisicos en la analgesia del parto normal. *Rev. esp. Obstet. Ginec.*, Valencia (1955) **14**, 289–301.
161. O. Floel, Schmerzlose Entbindung in der Privatpraxis. *Münch. med. Wschr.* (1921) 1623.
162. N. Fodor, The Trauma of Bearing. *Psychiat. Quart.* (1949) **23**, 59–70.
163. P. Foissac, *Rapports et Discussions de l'Académie Royale de Médecine sur le Magnétisme Animal.* J. B. Baillère, Paris (1833).
164. T. Fontan and Ch. Segard, *Eléments de Médecine Suggestive. Faits Cliniques.* O. Doin, Paris (1887).
165. C. S. Ford, *A Comparative Study of 'Human Reproduction'.* Yale University Publications in Anthropology, Yale Univ. Press, New Haven (1945) No. 32.
166. A. Forel, *Der Hypnotismus* 6th ed. Stuttgart (1911).
167. A. Forel, *1st International Congress of Experimental and Therapeutic Hypnotism* held in l'Hôtel-Dieu in Paris, 8–12, August (1889).
168. J. A. Fort, Extraction d'une loupe pendant le sommeil hypnotique sur un jeune homme de vingt ans. (153) 202–205. *Rev. Hypnot.*, Paris (1890) 142.
169. F. Fraipont and J. Delbœuf, Accouchement dans l'hypnotisme. *Rev. Hypnot.*, Paris, (1891) 289–298.
170. U. Franke, Die Hypnosegeburten des praktischen Arztes. *Dtsch. med. Wschr.* (1923) 1341–1342.
171. U. Franke, Amnesie und Anaesthesie bei der Hypnosegeburt. *Dtsch. med. Wschr.* (1924) 874–875.
172. L. Z. Freedman and V. S. Ferguson, The question of 'painless childbirth' in primitive cultures. *Amer. J. Orthopsychiat.* (1950) **20**, 363–372.
173. L. Z. Freedman, F. Redlich, L. D. Eron and E. Jackson, Training for childbirth: remembrance of labour. *Psychosom. Med.* (1952) 439–452.
174. S. Freud, Ein Fall von hypnotischer Heilung nebst Bemerkungen über die Entstehung hysterischer Symptome durch den Gegenwillen. *Z. Hypnot.* (1893) 102–107; 123–129.
175. S. Freud, Charcot. *Wien. med. Wschr.*, (1893) 1512–1520.
176. S. Freud, *On Origins of Psycho-Analysis.* Ed. Bonaparte, Freud and Kris.
177. S. Freud, *Autobiographical Study* (1935) trans. Mosbacher and Strachey (1954) Imago, Hogarth, London,
178. S. Freud, *Beyond the Pleasure Principle.* Hogarth, London (1922).
179. S. Freud, *Inhibitions, Symptoms and Anxiety.* Hogarth, London (1936).
180. A. A. Friedlaender, Hypnonarkose. *Münch. med. Wschr.* (1919) 1198–1199.
181. M. E. Fries, Mental hygiene in pregnancy, delivery and the puerperium. *Ment. Hyg.*, London (1941) **25**, 221–236.

182. J. FRIGYESI and O. MANSFIELD, Über den suggestiven Dämmerschlaf und andere Arten der 'schmerzlosen Geburt'. *Innsbruck Congress* (91) 320–324.
183. F. FROMM-REICHMANN, Perception of pain and some factors that modify it. *Problems of consciousness* (405) 112–122.
184. J. GAILLARD, *Pratique de l'Accouchement sans Douleur.* Maloine, Paris (1955).
185. J. GAILLARD, Technique de l'accouchement dirigé indolore; avec éducation psychique, respiratoire et neuro-musculaire. *Concours med.* (1955) **77**, 1611–1614.
186. N. L. GARMACHEVA, Physical conditions in painless childbirth. *Leningrad Congress* (89) 19–28.
187. M. GAVEL, Les aspects de l'accouchement psychoprophylactique dans les petits centres. *Bull. Féd. Soc. Gyn. Obst. franç.* (1956) **8**, 485–486.
188. W. GEISENDORF, Le comportement de la femme préparée à l'accouchement sans douleur, aspects psychosomatiques. *La Journée d'Études sur les Méthodes Psychologiques en Analgésie Obstétricale*, Paris, 7 April (1957).
189. B. GELB, *The A.B.C. of Natural Childbirth.* W. W. Norton, New York (1954).
190. S. GLASNER, A note on allusions to hypnosis in the Bible and Talmud. *J. Clin. and exp. Hypnosis* (1955) **3**, 34–39.
191. R. GOIRAND, A propos de 100 cas d'accouchements après préparation suivant la méthode psychoprophylactique. *Bull. Féd. Soc. Gyn. Obst. franç.* (1955) **7**, 55–58.
192. F. W. GOODRICH, *Natural Childbirth. A Manual for Expectant Parents.* Prentice-Hall, New York (1950).
193. F. W. GOODRICH and H. THOMS, A clinical study of natural childbirth. *Amer. J. Obstet. Gynec.* (1948) **56**, 875–883.
194. F. W. GOODRICH, Emotion in pregnancy and labour as related to natural childbirth. *Problems of Early Infancy* (906) Second Conference, 34–41.
195. T. V. GOURSTEIN, A case of obstetrical analgesia under hypnosis. *Vrach. Dyelo* (1931) **5–6**, 288–289.
196. A. M. GOURVITCH, On the role of the bulbar reticular formation in the mechanisms of consciousness. *J. Vyschei Nervnoi Deiatelnosti* (1956) **6**, 482–493.
197. GRANDALIANO, L. MOLLARD and ARLAUD, Resultats de la psychoprophylactie de l'accouchement. (A propos de 1000 cas). *Bull. Féd. Soc. Gyn. d'Obst.* (1956) **8**, 518–520.
198. DE GRANDCHAMPS, Accouchement en était de fascination, insensibilité complète pendant la période d'expulsion; régularisation des contractions, amnésie totale au réveil. *Gaz. Hôp., Paris*, (1889) 857–858.
199. J. GRASSET and J. DUMONT, Accouchement physiologiquement accéléré et à douleurs atténuées. *Concours méd.* (1955) **77**, 2361–2362.

200. J. Grasset and J. Dumont, Les orientations actuelles des techniques de l'analgésie obstétricale: les méthodes neuropsychiques. *Pr. méd.* (1954) **62,** 419–421.
201. Grassl, Zur Frage der schmerzlosen Geburt. *Münch. med. Wschr.* (1921) No. 44.
202. P. Greenacre, The biological economy of birth. *The Psycho-analytic Study of the Child,* Int. University Press, New York (1945) Vol. 1, 31–51.
203. H. S. Greer, Hypnotic analgesia in childbirth. *Med. J. Aust.* (1956) **43,** 819–820.
204. L. Gregoire, L'accouchement sans douleur. *Rev. méd. Liège* (1956) 428–432.
205. R. R. Grinker, Psychosomatic approach to anxiety. *Amer. J. Psychiat.* (1956) **113,** 443–447.
206. J. Grossman, Suggestion und Milchsekretion. *Z. Hypnot.* (1893) 71–72.
207. Dr. Gueckel, Suggestive Narkose: Psychotherapeutische Forderungen zur Narkose. *Münch. med. Wschr.* (1919) 1001–1002.
208. A. K. Gueorguievski, Concerning the use of hypnotic suggestion in obstetrical analgesia. *Bull. Univ. Nijni-Novogrod* (1930) 249–264.
209. G. B. Guerenstein, Hypnosis in obstetrics and gynaecology. *J. Akush i Jenskikh Bolezni* (1924) **35,** 235–240.
210. G. B. Guerenstein, Psychotherapy in obstetrics and gynaecology. *J. Akush i Jenskikh Bolezni* (1925) **36,** 671–678.
211. Guérineau, Observation d'hypnotisme dans un cas d'amputation de cuisse. *Gaz. Hôp., Paris,* (1859) 607–608.
212. G. Guillain, *J. M. Charcot (1825–1893), Sa Vie, son Oeuvre.* Masson & Co., Paris (1955).
213. A. C. Haddon, *Reports of the Cambridge Anthropological Expedition to Torres Straits.* Cambridge Univ. Press (1907) 6 vols.
214. K. E. Hagbarth and D. I. B. Kerr, Central influences on spinal afferent conduction. *J. Neurophysiol.* (1954) **17,** 295–307.
215. D. Hall and G. Mohr, Prenatal attitudes of primiparae: a contribution to the mental hygiene of pregnancy. *Ment. Hyg.* (1933) **17,** 226–234.
216. G. J. Hall, Modern changes in the attitude toward the pain of labour. *Med. J. Aust.* (1954) **41,** 289–291.
217. B. Hallauer, Die Hypnose in Gynaekologie und Geburtshilfe und die Narkohypnose. *Zbl. Gynäk.* (1922) 45, 1793–1808.
218. J. D. Hardy, H. G. Wolff and H. Goodell. *Pain Sensations and Reactions.* Williams and Wilkins, Baltimore. (1952).
219. F. Harlin, *Préparez-vous une Heureuse Maternité.* Les Presses d'aujourd'hui. Denoel, Paris (1951).
220. F. Havranek, Estimation des résultats de la préparation psychoprophylactique à l'accouchement sans douleur. *Prakt. Lek., Prague,* (1953) **33,** 116–118.

221. H. Heardman, *Physiotherapy in Obstetrics and Gynaecology (including Education for Childbirth)*. E. and S. Livingstone, Edinburgh (1951).
222. H. Heardman, *A Way to Natural Childbirth*. Williams and Wilkins, Baltimore (1948).
223. H. Heardman, *Relaxation and Exercise for Natural Childbirth*. E. and S. Livingstone, Edinburgh (1955).
224. H. Heberer, 50 Geburten in Hypnose. *Zbl. Gynäk.* (1922). 749–751.
225. R. Held, Névrose et grossesse: Quelques réflexions cliniques. *La Journée d'Études sur les Méthodes Psychologiques en Analgésie Obstétricale*, Paris, 7 April (1957).
226. R. Hellmann, Der psychische Faktor in der Geburtshilfe. *La Semaine Psychothérapique de Lindau* (1955) Georg. Thieme Stugart, 31–43.
227. R. Hellmann, Zur Psychologisierung der Geburtshilfe. *Zbl. Gynäk.* (1956) **78**, 1655–1671.
228. A. Hernandez Jimenez, La pratique de la méthode psychoprophylactique en clientèle privée. *La Journée d'Etudes sur les Méthodes Psychologiques en Analgésie Obstétricale*, Paris 7 April (1957).
229. R. Hernandez-Peon and H. Scherrer, Inhibitory influence of brain stem reticular formation upon synoptic transmission in trigeminal nucleus. *Fed. Proc.* (1955) **14**, 71.
230. R. Hernandez-Peon, H. Scherrer and M. Jouvet, Modification of electric activity in cochlear nucleus during 'attention' in unanaesthetized cats. *Science*, (1956) **123**, 331–332.
231. J. Hirst and T. Strousse, The origin of emotional factors in normal pregnant women. *Amer. J. med. Sci.* (1938) **196**, 95–98.
232. N. M. Holmer and S. H. Wassen, The complete MU-IGALA in picture writing. A native record of a cuna indian medicine song. Goteborg (1953).
233. J. Horsky, Conditions et déroulement de la préparation psychoprophylactique à la salle de travail. *Prakt. Lek., Prague.* (1953) **33**, 109–113.
234. L. Hrasko, Préparation psychoprophylactique à l'accouchement sans douleur. *Lekarsky Obzor. Bratislava* (1954) **3**, 221–224.
235. A. Hrdlicka, *Bull. Bur. Amer. Ethnol.* (1908) **34**. Quoted by True [539].
236. A. Hugelin, Analyse de l'inhibition d'un réflexe nociceptif (réflexe linguo-maxillaire) lors de l'activation du système réticulo-spinal dit 'facilitateur'. *C.R. Soc. Biol., Paris*, (1955) **149**, 1893–1898.
237. A. Hugelin, Étude comparée de l'activation du système réticulaire activateur ascendant et du système réticulaire facilitateur descendant. *C.R. Soc. Biol., Paris* (1955) **149**, 1963–1965.
238. A. Hugelin, Les bases physiologiques de la vigilance. *Encéphale* G. Doin, Paris (1956), **45**, 267–287.
239. I. I. Iakovlev, C. M. Lisovskaia and G. A. Shminke, Electrical activity of the cerebral cortex during preparation by the psychoprophylactic method. *Akush. Ginek.* (1954) **1**, 3–8.

240. IOFFE, Concerning hypnotherapy. *Dniepropetrovskij med. journal* (1928) No. 1–2, 70–75.
241. A. P. IOFFE, Psychotherapeutic hypnosuggestive practice in obstetrics. *Vrach. Dyelo* (1929) **11**, 747.
242. P. P. ISTOMINE and R. IA. CHLIFFER, Concerning psychotherapy and its biological worth during pregnancy and childbirth. *Psikhoterapia, Kharkov* (1930) 319–326.
243. A. G. IVANOV-SMOLENSKI, The interactions of the first and second signalling systems in some physiological and some pathological states. *Setchenov J. Physiol.* (1949) **36**, French transl. *La Raison, Paris* (1951) **1**, 54–67.
244. A. G. IVANOV-SMOLENSKI, *A Summary of the Physiopathology of Higher Nervous Activity.* Medquiz, Moscow (1952), 2nd ed. German transl. *Grundzuege der Pathophysiologie der hoeheren Nerventaetigkeit.* U. Bauer, Academie Verlag, Berlin (1954).
245. E. JACOBSON, *Progressive Relaxation.* Chicago Univ. Press, Chicago. (1938).
246. E. JACOBSON, Relaxation methods in labour: a critique of current technique in natural childbirth. *Amer. J. Obstet. Gynec.* (1954) **67**, 1035–1048.
247. P. JANET, *Psychological Healing.* Transl. PAUL. Allen & Unwin (1925). 3 vols.
248. P. JANET, *La Médecine Psychologique.* Flammarion, Paris (1923).
249. C. T. JAVERT and J. D. HARDY, Influence of analgesics on pain intensity during labor (with a note on 'natural childbirth'). *Anesthesiology* (1951) **12**, 189–215.
250. C. JEANSON, *Principes et Pratique de l'Accouchement sans Douleur.* Seuil, Paris (1954).
251. I. N. JELOKHOVZSEVA, An objective study of the pain of childbirth by plethysmography. *Leningrad Congress* (89) 161–168.
252. W. JOCHELSON, The Yukaghir and the youkaghirized tungus. Vol. XIII of the *Mem. Amer. Mus. Nat. Hist.* which constitutes, at the same time, Vol. IX Part I of the Jesup North Pacific Expedition. New York and Leiden (1910).
253. P. JOIRE, De l'emploi de l'analgésie hypnotique dans les accouchements. *Rev. Hypnot., Paris* (1899) **13**, 39–59.
254. DE JONG, *1st Int. Congr. Experimental and Therapeutic Hypnotism*, held at the Hôtel-Dieu in Paris, 8–12 August 1889. O. Doin, Paris (1889) p. 205.
255. I. F. JORDANIA, Five years of psychoprophylactic preparation for childbirth. *Kiev Congress* (90) 38–47.
256. I. F. JORDANIA, Experience of the psychoprophylactic regime in a maternity unit. *Akush. Ginek* (1952), 4 *Cahiers de Médecine Soviétique*, (1953) 171–180. (French transl.).
257. Dr. JOURNÉE, Grossesse, hypnose pendant la première partie du travail. *Rev. Hypnot., Paris*, (1891) 18–20.

236   PSYCHOSOMATIC METHODS IN PAINLESS CHILDBIRTH

258. La Journée d'Etudes sur les Methodes Psychologique en Analgésie Obstétricale, Paris, 7 April (1957).
259. M. JOUVET, Aspects neurophysiologiques de quelques mécanismes du comportement. *J. Psychol. norm. path.* (1956) **53,** 141–162.
260. I. M. KALACHNIK, Concerning the use of hypnosis during pregnancy and labour. *Odessaer med. Zh.* (1927) No. 8–10, 85–89.
261. F. D. KARTCHNER, A study of the emotional reactions during labour. *Amer. J. Obstet. Gynec.* (1950) **60,** 19–29.
262. F. A. KATCHAN and G. G. BELOZERSKI, Obstetrical analgesia by hypnosis and suggestion. *Sborn. tsent. nauch.-issled. akouch-guinek. Inst. Leningrad,* (1940) **6,** 19–89.
263. K. KEKTCHEEV and F. A. SYROVATKO, Concerning interoceptive stimulations in women. *Akush. Ginek.* (1939) 5.
264. G. G. KHETCHINACHVILI, Reflex reaction of the vessels through excitation of the uterine receptors in pregnant and parturient women. *Bull. Eksp. Biol. i Med.,* (1952) No. 11.
265. G. O. KINGSBURY, Accouchement pendant le sommeil hypnotique. *Rev. Hypnot.,* Paris (1891), 298–300.
266. N. IU. KIRITCHENKO, *Psychoprophylactic Preparation of Pregnant Women for Childbirth.* (*Course for the use of tutor-midwives*). Cosmedizdat of the S.S.R. of the Ukraine (1957).
267. F. KIRSTEIN, Ueber Hypnosegeburten und Hypnonarkosen. *Zbl. Gynäk.* (1922), **21,** 843–850.
268. KISLOV, Quoted by VELVOSKI [558].
269. H. KLEIN, H. POTTER and R. DYK, *Anxiety in Pregnancy and Childbirth.* Psychosomatic Med. Monograph. Paul Hoeber, Inc., New York (1950).
270. E. KLEMPERER, Hypnotherapy. *J. nerv. ment. Dis.* **106** (1947) No. 2, 176–185.
271. M. KLINE and H. GUZE, Self-hypnosis in childbirth: A clinical evaluation of a patient-conditioning program. *J. Clin. exp. Hypnosis,* (1955) **3,** 142–147.
272. M. G. KLOOSTERMAN, L'aspect psychologique de la prophylaxie des douleurs de l'accouchement. *Brux. med.* (1955) 35–28, 1389–1400.
273. A. A. KOGAN, Suggestive method of obstetrical analgesia. *Akush. Ginek.* (1947) 50.
274. M. I. KOGANOV, Painless childbirth through suggestion without prior hypnotic preparation. *Akush. Ginek.* (1951) **11,** 31–34.
275. H. KOGERER, Die posthypnotische Geburtsanalgesie. *Wien. klin. Wschr.* (1922) 513–17, 538–540, 558–561.
276. H. KOGERER, Bemerkungen zur arbeit, Zum kapitel hypnosegeburten vom F. Schultze-Rhonhof in N 21 dieses zentralblattes. *Zbl. Gynäk.* (1923) **47,** 889.
277. V. I. KONSTANTINOV, Theory and practice of psychoprophylactic preparation for childbirth. *Kiev Congress* (90) 11–17.
278. Z. A. KOPIL-LEVINA, The method of obstetrical analgesia through

verbal suggestion. K. I. Platonov. *Problems of Psychotherapy in Obstetrics*, Kharkov (1940) 34–65.
279. Z. A. KOPIL-LEVINA and M. I. LINIEVITCH, Two cases of verbal analgesia in difficult childbirths, p. 67–72 in PLATONOV *Problems of Psychotherapy in Obstetrics*, Kharkov (1940).
280. B. K. KORABELNIK and D. I. DARON, Use of the psychoprophylactic method in a maternity unit. *Leningrad Congress* (89) 60–64.
281. A. D. KOUDACHEV, Experience of hypnosis in obstetrics and gynaecology. *Kazansk. med. Zh.* (1927) **12**, 1253–1263.
282. W. KROENIG and L. SCHOENHOLZ, Über den medikamentösen und hypnotischen Dämmerschlaf in der Gebursthilfe. *Mschr. Geburtsh. Gynäk.* (1923) **61**, 16–179.
283. W. S. KROGER, Hypnotherapy in Obstetrics and Gynecology. *J. Clin. and exp. Hypnosis* (1953) **1**, 61–70.
284. W. S. KROGER, 'Natural childbirth': Is Read's method of 'natural childbirth' waking hypnotism? *Brit. J. Med. Hypnot.* (1953) 1–15.
285. W. S. KROGER, Psychosomatic aspects of obstetrics and gynecology, *Obstetrics and Gynecology*, N.Y., (1954) **3**, 504–516.
286. W. S. KROGER and S. C. FREED, *Psychosomatic Gynecology: Including Problems of Obstetrical Care*. W. B. Saunders, Philadelphia (1951).
287. W. S. KROGER and S. T. DE LEE, The use of the hypnoidal state as an amnestic, analgesic and anesthetic agent in obstetrics. *Amer. J. Obstet. Gynec.* (1943) **46**, 655–661.
288. W. S. KROGER and S. T. DE LEE, Hypnoanesthesia for Caesarean section and hysterectomy. *J. Amer. med. Ass.* (1957) **163**, 442–444.
289. L. S. KUBIE, Psychosomatic Aspects of Educated Childbirth, ed. H. B. DAVIDSON [114]. *N.Y. St. J. Med.* (1953) **6**, 2508–2509.
290. M. LACOMME, Avant-propos. *Maternité* (1954) **3**, 91–97.
291. Ch. LAFONTAINE, *L'Art de Magnétiser ou le Magnétisme Animal*. 3rd ed. Baillère, Paris (1860).
292. M. D. LAIRD and M. HOGAN, An elective program on preparation for childbirth at the Sloane Hospital for Women, May 1951 to June 1953. *Amer. J. Obstet. Gynec.* (1956) **72**, 641–647.
293. F. LAMAZE, L'expérience française de l'accouchement sans douleur. *Bull. Cerc. Claude Bernard* (1954) **8**, 2–5.
294. F. LAMAZE, Avant-propos. *Revue de la Nouvelle Médecine* (1954) **3**, 5–8.
295. F. LAMAZE, Les maternités soviétiques et l'accouchement sans douleur. *Revue de la Nouvelle Médecine* (1955) **5**, 61–66.
296. F. LAMAZE, La suppression de la douleur liée à la contraction de l'utérus en travail. *Int. Congr. Gynaecology and Obstetrics at La Havane, Cuba*, 4–10 December 1955. *Revue de la Nouvelle Médecine*, Paris (1956) **7**, 61–84.
297. F. LAMAZE, *Qu'est-ce que l'Accouchement sans Douleur par la Méthode Psychoprophylactique. Ses Principes, sa Réalisation, ses Résultats*. Savoir et Connaître, Paris (1956).
298. F. LAMAZE and P. VELLAY, L'accouchement sans douleur par la

méthode psychophysique. Premiers résultats portant sur 500 cas. *Gaz. méd. Fr.* (1952) **59**, 1445–1460.

299. F. LAMAZE and P. VELLAY, Considération sur l'accouchement sans douleur par la méthode psychophysique (Travail de la Maternité de la Polyclinique du Métallurgiste.) *Revue de la Nouvelle Médecine*, (1953) **1**, 71–77.

300. F. LAMAZE and P. VELLAY, Application de la méthode psychoprophylactique dans quelques cas particuliers: chez les pulmonaires, chez les cardiaques, dans les sièges et applications de forceps Suzor sans anesthésie. *Congr. Féd. Soc. Gyn. Obstet. franç. Bruxelles*, 22–26 September (1955).

301. F. LAMAZE, P. VELLAY and H. HERSILIE, Considérations sur la technique de l'accouchement sans douleur. *Revue de la Nouvelle Médecine* (1954) **3**, 63–68.

302. F. LAMAZE, P. VELLAY and H. HERSILIE, Essai d'interprétation des causes d'échec. *Revue de la Nouvelle Médecine* (1954) **3**, 129–140.

303. F. LAMAZE, P. VELLAY and H. HERSILIE, Réponses à quelques questions. *Revue de la Nouvelle Médecine*, (1954) **3**, 125–128.

304. F. LAMAZE, P. VELLAY, H. HERSILIE, H. ANGELERGUES and A. BOURREL, Expérience pratiquée à la maternité du Centre Pierre Rouquès sur la méthode d'accouchement sans douleur par la psychoprophylaxie. *Bull Acad. nat. Méd.* (1954) **138**, 52–58.

305. F. LAMAZE, and P. VELLAY, Cinq ans d'expérimentation de la méthode psychoprophylactique d'accouchement sans douleur. *La Journée d'Etudes sur les Méthodes Psychologiques en Analgésie Obstétricale*, 7 April 1957.

306. F. LAMAZE and B. MULDVORF, Les aspects psychologiques, psychothérapiques, et les incidences sociales de l'accouchement sans douleurs. *Bull. Féd. Soc. Gyn. Obstet. franç.* (1956) **8**, 549–558.

307. J. LAMBERT, A propos d'un récent débat sur l'accouchement sans douleur. *Sem. Hôp., Paris* (1954) **30**, 2433–2436.

308. G. LANGEVIN-DROGUET, Préparation physique et psychologique à l'accouchement. *Maternité* (1954) **3**, 122–128.

309. P. LANTUEJOUL and R. MERGER, La douleur de l'accouchement et sa psychoprophylaxie. *Sem. Hôp., Paris* (1954) **30**, 2198–2202.

310. P. LANTUEJOUL, L'accouchement normal, naturel ou forcé? *Hôpital* (1955) **43**, 290–291.

311. J. M. LARRIBÈRE, Premières observations d'accouchement sans douleur. *Bull. Féd. Soc. Gyn. Obstet. franç.* (1954) **6**, 54–55.

312. J. LASSNER, Eléments d'une anesthésiologie. *Anésth. Analg.* (1953) **10**, 184–192.

313. J. LASSNER, Hypnose et anesthésie. *Anésth. Analg.* (1954) **11**, 789–807.

314. K. LASZLO, E. GYULA and I. LASZLO, Childbirth among woman atheletes. *Orvosi Hetilap* (1957) **98** No. 7–8, 153–158.

315. M. LECOMTE, L'accouchement psychoprophylactique. *Revue du Praticien, Paris* (1955) **5**, 21.

316. B. LEE, The analgesic effects of rapid and forcible respiration. *Philadelphia Medical Times.* Philadelphia (1880) **10**, 498–500.
317. G. LE LORIER, L'analgésie obstétricale. *Maternité, Paris* (1954) **3**, 98–122.
318. G. LE LORIER, Avant-propos. En coll. avec le Dr. Comet et Mlle Leclerc: Théorie, pratique et résultats de l'accouchement sans douleur. *Maternité, Paris* (1956), 139–163.
319. LE MENANT DE CHESNAIS, Avantage du sommeil suggéré contre certaines douleurs et en particulier contre celles de l'accouchement. *Rev. Hypnot., Paris* (1894), 324–330.
320. A. LEONARD, *De l'hystérie Pendant la Grossesse et le Travail de l'Accouchement.* Thesis (1886–87), Librairie Ollier-Henry.
321. F. LEPAGE and G. LANGEVIN-DROGUET, A propos de la préparation physique et psychique des femmes à l'accouchement. *Pr. méd.* (1955) **63**, 549–551.
322. F. LEPAGE and G. LANGEVIN-DROGUET, Préparation à l'accouchement suivant la méthode du Dr. Read. *La Journée d'Études sur les Méthodes Psychologiques en Analgésie Obstétricale, Paris,* 7 April 1957.
323. R. LERICHE, *Bases de la Chirurgie Physiologique. Essai sur la Vie Végétative des Tissues.* Masson & Co., Paris (1955).
324. J. LESINSKI, *Prophylaxie des Douleurs de l'Accouchement.* State Medical Editions, Warsaw (1956).
325. Cl. LEVY-STRAUSS, Sorciers et psychanalyse. *Le courier de l'Unesco* (1956) No. 7–8, 808–810.
326. I. B. LEVIT and F. I. RABINOVITCH, Psychoprophylaxis of the pains of childbirth. *Akush. Ginek.* (1955) **1**, 33–36.
327. J. LEVY, La préparation psychoprophylactic à l'accouchement *Cahiers d'anesthesiologie*, **4**, (1957) Nos. 413–425.
328. L. LICHTSCHEIN, Hypnotism in pregnancy and labor. *Medical News,* New York (1898) **73**, 295–298.
329. A. A. LIEBAULT, *Du Sommeil et des États Analogues Considéré surtout au Point de Vue de l'Action du Moral sur le Physique.* Masson and Son, Paris (1866).
330. A. A. LIEBAULT, Anesthésie par suggestion *Journal du Magnetisme* (1885) 64–67.
331. J. LIÉGEOIS, *De la Suggestion et du Somnambulisme dans leurs Rapports avec la Jurisprudence et la Médecine Légale.* O. Doin, Paris (1889).
332. B. LIEGNER, Die Suggestivbehandlung in der Fraunheilkunde. *Zbl. Gynäk.* (1922) No. 3, 89–92.
333. H. LOHMER, 5 Jahre Erfahrungen mit der modifizierten Readschen Methode der angstfreien Geburt. *Med. Klinik, Munich* (1955) **50**, 1828–1830.
334. A. IOU. LOURIE, The practice of psychoprophylactic preparation for childbirth in the Obstetrical Institutions of the Ukrainian S.S.R. *Kiev Congress* (90) 29–33.

335. A. LOYSEL, *Recueil d'Opérations Chirurgicales Pratiquées sur des Sujets Magnétisés.* Beaufort and Lecauf, Cherbourg (1846).
336. LUGEOL, Accouchement dans le sommeil hypnotique. *Mém. Bull. Soc. méd. chir.*, *Bordeaux* (1894) 552–55.
337. K. H. LUKAS, Readsche Geburtserleichterung in der Klinik. *Med. Klinik, Munich* (1954) **49,** 1720–1721.
338. J. LUYS, Accouchement en état de fascination; amnésie complète au réveil. *Rev. Hypnot., Paris* (1890) 321–323.
339. J. LUYS, Deux cas nouveaux d'accouchement sans douleur. *Rev. Hypnot., Paris* (1890), 49–55.
340. J. LUYS, Modifications circulatoires survenues dans l'aréole du sein chez une femme hypnotisable, sous l'influence d'une suggestion. *Rev. Hypnot., Paris* (1890) 215–217.
341. R. LYONNET, Propos sur les méthodes de préparation et de direction non médicamenteuse de l'accouchement. *Lyon Méd.* (1956) **88,** 9–19.
342. M. MABILIE and S. RAMADIER, Anesthésie chirurgicale par suggestion post-hypnotique. *Rev. Hypnot., Paris* (1886–1887), 111–112.
343. J. MADDERS, Physiotherapy and antenatal care. III. Training for natural childbirth; the mental aspect. *Physiotherapy, Lond.* (1955) **41,** 173–176.
344. J. MALAGUTI, *Sur les Difficultés d'une Application Rigoureuse de la Méthode Psychoprophylactique en Milieu Hospitalier à Propos d'une Serie de 100 Accouchements Conduits selon cette Technique.* Thesis, Paris (1955), No. 501.
345. P. MALCOVATI, Mon expérience de psychoprophylaxie obstétricale. *La Journée d'Études sur les Méthodes Psychologiques en Analgésie Obstétricale,* 7 April, 1957.
346. A. J. MANDY, R. FARKAS, E. SCHER and T. E. MANDY, The natural childbirth illusion. *Sth. med. J., Birmingham* (1951) **44,** 527–534.
347. A. J. MANDY, T. E. MANDY, H. FARKAS and E. SCHER, Is natural childbirth natural? *Psychosom. Med.* (1952) **14,** 432–438.
348. E. M. MARSH, W. G. MOORE and A. M. VOLLMER, *Your Baby is Born,* Accommodation Letter Shop, San Francisco (1949).
349. G. MARTIUS, Schmerzlinderung unter der Geburt. *Dtsch. med. Wschr.* (1956) **81,** 1547–1551.
350. A. A. MASON, Surgery under hypnosis. *Anaesthesia* (1955) **10,** 295–299.
351. G. F. MATVEEV, Narcosis and hypnosis during pregnancy and labour. *Communication to the 8th Congress of the Society of Russian doctors (Pirogov)* (1902), Summary in WIAZEMSKY [576].
352. R. MAUREL, *La Méthode Psychoprophylactique d'Accouchement sans Douleur et la Place qui lui Revient parmi les Méthodes d'Analgesie Obstétricale.* Thesis, Paris (1954), No. 615.
353. M. MAYER, L'enseignement de la puériculture en maternité. (Une expérience hospitalière d'éducation psychologique et pratique de

puériculture pré et post-natale). *Sem. Hôp., Paris* (*Annales de Pédiatrie*), (1955), **31**.
354. M. Mayer, La méthode de l'accouchement naturel ('Accouchement sans douleur') en pratique hospitalière privée. (Ses principes son mode d'application et ses résultats). *A.I.M.F., Paris*, (1955) **33**, 9–31; **34**, 7–55.
355. M. Mayer, La douleur dans l'accouchement. *Conférence at the Collège Philosophique, Paris*, 22 February (1956).
356. M. Mayer, *Heidelberg Symposium*, 21 September (1956).
357. M. Mayer and J. Bonhomme, La méthode de l'accouchement naturel. Son utilisation en pratique hospitalière. *Vie méd.* (1953) **34**, 751–766.
358. M. Mayer and A. Morali-Daninos, Accouchement naturel et la psychosomatique. *La Journée d'Études sur les Méthodes Psychologiques en Analgésie Obstétricale, Paris*, 7 April, 1957.
359. M. Mead, *Male and Female. A Study of the Sexes in a Changing World*. Mentor books, New York (1955).
360. Mme Medeiros, *O Método Psicoprofiláctico das Dores do Parto: Experiencia Pessoal*. Dissertation, Faculty of Medicine, Lisbon. October (1956).
361. W. R. Merz, Einfluss der gymnastischen und psychischen Geburtsverbereitung auf wehenzahl und Geburtskauer. *Gynaecologia* (1956) **142**, 361–368.
362. F. A. Mesmer, *Mémoire sur la Découverte du Magnétisme Animal*. P. F. Didot le Jeune, Paris (1779).
363. Mesnet, De l'accouchement dans le somnambulisme provoqué. *Rev. Hypnot., Paris* (1888), 33–42.
364. Mesnet, Cystocèle vaginale, opération faite dans le sommeil hypnotique. *Bull. Acad. Méd. Paris* (1889) **22**, 92–102.
365. R. Meylan, L'accouchement sans douleur. *Rev. méd. Suisse rom.* (1955) **75**, 505–509.
366. A. M. Michael, Hypnosis in childbirth. *Brit. Med. J.* (1952), 734–737.
367. C. Mieville, A propos de l'accouchement dit sans douleur. *Praxis*, (1955) **44**, 988–990.
368. H. L. Miller, F. E. Flannery and D. Bell, Education for childbirth in private practice; 450 consecutive cases. *Amer. J. Obstet. Gynec.* (1952) **63**, 792–799.
369. Miloslavski, Quoted by Velvovski [558].
370. A. Moll. *Der Hypnotismus* 5th Ed. Berlin (1924).
371. J. C. Moloney, The cornelian corner and its rationale. *First Conference*, (406), 17–26.
372. P. Monjardino, Parto dem dor? Parto sem medo? Parto natural? *J. Méd. Porto* (1955) **26**, 645–658.
373. E. Montgomery, The physical therapist in the obstetric team. *Physiotherapy, Lond.* (1956) **42**, 211–215.
374. G. Moruzzi and H. W. Magoun, Brain stem reticular formation

and activation of the EEG. *Electroenceph. clin. neurophysiol.* (1949) **1**, 455–473.
375. A. C. MOTSAK, Quoted by VELVOVSKI [558].
376. J. P. MURPHY and E. GELLHORN, The influence of hypothalamic stimulation on cortically induced movements and on action potentials of the cortex. *J. Neurophysiol.* **8**, 339–364.
377. P. MURPHY, Expectant mothers organize for natural childbirth. *Amer. J. Nurs.* (1956) **56**, 1298–1301.
378. M. NASSAUER, Die Schmerzlose Geburt. *Münch. med. Wschr.* (1921) **42**, 1364–1366.
379. G. NEWBOLD, The use of hypnosis in obstetrics. *Brit. J. med. Hypnot.* (1949), 36–38.
380. G. NEWBOLD, The importance of hypnotism in midwifery. *Brit. J. med. Hypnot.* (1950) **2**, 2–6.
381. G. NEWBOLD, Hypno-relaxation classes in ante-natal clinics. *Brit. J. med. Hypnot.*, (1951) **2**, 44–47.
382. G. NEWBOLD, Hypnosis and home confinements. *Brit. J. med. Hypnot.*, (1953) **5**, 28–33.
383. A. P. NICOLAIEV, Hypnosis in obstetrics and gynaecology. *Vrach. Gaz.* (1924) No. 19–20, 417–419.
384. A. P. NICOLAIEV, Hypnosis in obstetrics and in surgery. *Kazans. med. Zh.* (1926) **1**, 50–54.
385. A. P. NICOLAIEV, Theory and practice of hypnosis from the physiological point of view. *Kiev Congress*, (90).
386. A. P. NICOLAIEV, Some questions concerning the principles of obstetrical analgesia. *Obezbolivanie Rodov. Papers given at 2nd Conf. Obstetricians and Gynaecologists of the Donetz region, Stalino* (1936), 50–59.
387. A. P. NICOLAIEV, The suggestive method in obstetrical analgesia. *Instruction on obstetrical analgesia, Stalino* (1936), 135–164.
388. A. P. NICOLAIEV, Fundamental principles and methods of painless childbirth. *Leningrad Congress* (89), 29–37.
389. A. P. NICOLAIEV, Conclusion. *Leningrad Congress* (89), 175–178.
390. A. P. NICOLAIEV, The theoretical basis of the psychoprophylaxis of the pain of childbirth. *Akush. Ginek.* (1952), French transl. *Revue de la Médecine Nouvelle*, (1953) **1**, 61–69.
391. A. P. NICOLAIEV, The theory of I. P. Pavlov on the autonomic nervous system, a scientific basis for resolving the practical tasks in obstetrics and gynaecology. *J. Vyschei Nervnoi Deiatelnosti*, T.I. (1951) **5**, 667–681. French transl. *Cahiers de Médecine Soviétique* (1953) **1**, 153–170.
392. A. P. NICOLAIEV, *Theory and Practice of Obstetrical Analgesia.* Medguiz, Moscow (1953).
393. A. P. NICOLAIEV, Methodological problems of the psychoprophylactic preparation for childbirth. *Kiev Congress* (90), 17–21.
394. A. P. NICOLAIEV, Essential problems in the application of the

physiological teachings of Pavlov in obstetrics and gynaecology *Akouch. i. Guinek* **5** (1957) 42–57.
395. P. P. NIKOULINE, The influence of psychoprophylactic analgesia on the adrenaline and acetylcholine content of the blood. *Akush. Ginek.* (1952), 10–15.
396. W. C. W. NIXON, Foreword to HEARDMAN [221].
397. W. C. W. NIXON, Natural Childbirth. *L'Enfant. Oeuvre Nationale de l'Enfance, Bruxelles.* Numéro consacré aux travaux du Congr. pour l'études de la mortalité périnatale (1953) **5**, 235–254.
398. W. C. W. NIXON, Psychosomatic preparation for childbirth. *Proc. Roy. Soc. Med.* (1954), 395–387.
399. I. NOGUEIRA, Parto natural: fundamentos e técnica. *J. Méd. Porto* (1955), **6**.
400. NORDMAN, Accouchement sans douleur à Genève [4].
401. A. NOTTER, La méthode dite d'accouchement naturel de Read. *Bull. Féd. Soc. Gyn. Obstet. franç. Paris* (1952) **4**, 944–946.
402. A. NOTTER, La méthode dite d'accouchement sans douleurs par préparation psychique et physique. *Bull. Féd. Soc. Gyn. Obstet. franç., Paris* (1954) **6**, 73–74.
403. A. NOTTER and G. EGRON, L'accouchement psychophysique involontaire des tuberculeuses pulmonaires en traitement (A propos de 523 observations des années 1950 à 1954). *Gynéc. et Obstet.* (1956) **55**, 87–99.
404. A. NOTTER, Intérêt des données numériques de la pneumospirométrie dans la préparation psychophysiothérapique des gestantes à l'accouchement (1243 observations). *La Journée d'Études sur les Méthodes Psychologiques en Analgésie Obstétricale, Paris*, 7 April 1957.
405. VON OETTINGEN, Zur Frage der Schmerzlosen Geburt. *Münch. med. Wschr.* (1921) **51**, 1654–1655.
406. OUDET, *Bull. de l'Acad. Royale de Méd.* (1836/37), 343–347. J. B. Baillère, Paris.
407. A. OWNE-FLOOD, Hypnosis in anaesthesiology. J. SCHNECK *Hypnosis in Medicine*, Springfield (1953), 89–100.
408. I. P. PAVLOV, Works. *Academy of Science of the U.S.S.R.* (1951). 6 vols.
409. A. T. PCHONIK, The role of the cerebral cortex in the production of painful cutaneous sensations. *Probl. Kortiko-Vistzeralnoi Patolog.* Edit. Akad. Med. Nauk S.S.S.R., Moscow (1949), 33–35.
410. A. T. PCHONIK, *The Cerebral Cortex and the Receptive Function of the Organisms.* Moscow (1952) German transl. *Hirnrinde und rezeptorische Funktion des Organismus*, Akademie Verlag, Berlin (1956).
411. F. PEETERS, Étude clinique de l'emploi du R 875 en obstétrique. *La Presse Medicale*, (1958) **66**, No. 1, 8–9.
412. L. H. PETIT, L'anesthésie par la respiration rapide et l'hypnotisme *L'Encéphale*, (1881) 856–858.

413. M. A. PETROV-MASLAKOV, Experience in the application of psychoprophylactic preparation for labour. *Kiev Congress*, 90 62–66.
414. M. A. PETROV-MASLAKOV and R. A. ZATCHEPITZKI, The use of the method of painless childbirth on a large scale. *Cahiers de Médecine Soviétique* (1954) **2,** 49–56.
415. M. A. PETROV-MASLAKOV and R. A. ZATCHEPITZKI, *Psychoprophylaxis of the Pains of Childbirth*. Medguiz, Moscow (1953).
416. H. PIERON, La psychophysiologie générale de la douleur. *Proc. Pap. 13th Int. Congr. Psychol. Stockholm* (1951), 92–108.
417. H. PIGEAUD, L'accouchement à douleurs atténuées. *Progr. méd. Paris* (1954) **82,** 379–380.
418. H. PIGEAUD and A. NOTTER, Préparation psychophysiothérapique à l'accouchement dirigé (Organisme des séances préparatoires en Milieu Hospitalier). *Pr. méd.* (1956) **64,** 481–482.
419. H. PIGEAUD, R. GARMIER, R. HEUGHEBAERT and J. P. S. HOTTE, Premiers résultats de l'application des méthodes psychophysiothérapiques préparatoires à l'accouchement. *Rev. franç. Gynéc. Obstet.* (1956) **51,** 147–152.
420. A. PITRES, Anesthésie chirurgicale par suggestion. *J. Méd. Bordeaux*, (1886), 502–503.
421. K. I. PLATONOV, On the role of suggestion and hypnosis in obstetrics and gynaecology. *Akush Ginek.* (1927), 750–752. (7th Congress of Obstetricians and Gynaecologists of the U.S.S.R.).
422. K. I. PLATONOV, *Speech, a Physiological and Therapeutic Factor*. Kharkov (1930).
423. K. I. PLATONOV, Psychological factors in obstetrical analgesia. *Akush Ginek.* (1937), 93–99.
424. K. I. PLATONOV, Psychoprophylactic obstetrical analgesia in the light of Pavlovian theory. *Vrach. Dyelo* (1950), 1079–1082.
425. K. I. PLATONOV, *Suggestion and Hypnosis in the Light of the Writings of I. P. Pavlov*. Medguiz, Moscow (1951).
426. K. I. PLATONOV, Psychoprophylactic method of obstetrical analgesia. *Leningrad Congress* (89), 38–41.
427. K. I. PLATONOV, La parole en tant que facteur physiologique et thérapeutique. [558], lecture 2; French transl. *Commissions de Gynécologie, Obstétrique et de Neuropsychiatrie, France–U.R.S.S.* (1955).
428. K. I. PLATONOV and I. Z. VELVOVSKI, On the use of hypnosis in surgery, obstetrics and gynaecology. *Vrach. Dyelo* (1924), 353–356.
429. K. I. PLATONOV and M. V. CHESTOPAL, Suggestion and hypnosis in obstetrics and gynaecology. *Gos. Iz. d'Ukraine* (1925).
430. V. A. PLOTITCHER, [558] Lectures 9, 10, 11 and 12.
431. PORAK, Hypnotisme provoqué pendant la grossesse et le début du travail. Action de la compression des ovaires. Dédoublement de la personnalité. LEONARD [320] p. 74.
432. J. C. PORTNUFF, The trained obstetrical patient. *Amer. J. Obstet. Gynec.* (1954) **67,** 268–272.

433. G. S. POSTOLNIK, Experience in the use of hypnosis and suggestion in obstetrics. *J. Akouch. i Jenskikh Bolezni* (1930) **41**, 73–82.
434. A. B. PREISSMAN and ESSENOVA OGOULBOSTAN, Some details of psychoprophylactic preparation for childbirth in the Turkomenian S.S.R. *Kiev Congress*, (90), 66–67.
435. H. J. PRILL, Methoden psychischer Gevurtsschemerzerleichterung. *Geburtsh. Gynäk.* (1956) 211–229.
436. E. PRITZL, Un accouchement dans l'hypnose. *Rev. Hypnot., Paris*, (1886/87), 157–158. *Wien. med. Wschr.* (1885), 1365–1368.
437. Problems of consciousness. *Transactions of the First Conference sponsored by Josiah Macy Jr. Foundation* 20–21 March (1950) Ed. ABRAMSON (H). Corlies, Macy and Co., New York (1951).
438. Problems of Early Infancy. *Transactions of the First Conference* (1947), *Transactions of the Second Conference* (1948), *Josiah Macy Jr. Foundation*, New York.
439. PRONIAIEVA, Quoted by VELVOVSKI [558].
440. M. PRUDENT, *Les Causes d'Échec de la Méthode de l'Accouchement Naturel*. Thesis, (1956), No. 1004.
441. Marquis de PUYSÉGUR, *Mémoires pour Servir à l'Histoire et à l'Établissement du Magnétisme Animal*. 3rd ed. J. G. Dentu, Paris (1820).
442. K. I. PYRSKII, The problem of psychotherapy in obstetrics and gynaecology. *J. Akouch. i. Jenskikh Bolezni* (1927), **2**, 248–263.
443. QUICHON, Note sur l'application de la méthode psychoprophylactique en accouchement. *Gaz. méd. Fr.* (1956) **63**, 1195–1196.
444. J. RAEFLER, Die Hypnose in der Gynaekologie. *Zbl. Gyn.* 1921. No. 36. 1274–1278.
445. J. RAEFLER and FR. SCHULTZE-RHONHOF, Die Hypnose bei vaginalen Kursuntersuchungen *Zbl. Gyn.* 1921, No. 36, 1270–1273.
446. B. B. RAGINSKY, Mental suggestion as an aid in anesthesia. *Anesthesiology*, (1948) 9, 472–480.
447. G. RAIMBAULT, *L'accouchement Naturel: mise en Application à la Maternité St.-Antoine, Resultats Subjectifs et Objectifs, Intérêt d'un Approche Psychosomatique*. Thesis, Paris (1956).
448. S. RAMON CAJAL, Hypnotic suggestion in labour. *Brit. med. J.* (1889), 1053.
449. O. RANK, *Trauma of Birth* (Int. Lib. of Psychology, Philos and Scientific Method) Harcourt (1929).
450. S. G. RANSOM, L'analgésie obstétricale, *Brux. méd.* (1956) **36**, 121–131.
451. D. RAPAPORT, *Emotions and Memory*, 2nd ed. Int Univ. Press, New York (1950).
452. D. RAPAPORT, Perception of pain and some factors that modify it [437], 103–122.
453. RAPPORT, Second de la Commission nommée par le Gouvernement pour examiner les opérations chirurgicales faites par le Doct. J. Esdaile sur des malades soumis à l'influence d'un agent supposé,

dit mesmérique. (Hôpital magnétique de Calcutta). DU POTET [140] 597–606.
454. J. RAVINA, P. DEVRAIGNE, S. TSOULADZE and J. COENCA, La psychoprophylaxie de la douleur dans l'accouchement. *Sem. Hôp., Paris* (1954) **30**, 2202–2210.
455. I. IA. RAZDOLSKI, Problème de la douleur en clinique. *Leningrad Congress* (89), 9–18.
456. G. D. READ, *Natural Childbirth*. Wm. Heinemann, Lond. (1933).
457. G. D. READ, *Revelation of Childbirth*. Heinemann, Lond. Also appearing in the U.S.A. as *Childbirth without Fear*. Harper Bros., New York, (1944).
458. G. D. READ, *The Birth of a Child*. Wm. Heinemann. London (1947).
459. G. D. READ, An outline of the Conduct of Physiological Labor. *Amer. J. Obstet. Gynec.* (1947) **54**, 702–710.
460. G. D. READ, The discomforts of childbirth. *Brit. med. J.* (1949) **1**, 651.
461. G. D. READ, Observations on a series of labours. *Lancet* (1949), 721–736.
462. G. D. READ, The relief of pain in labour. *West. J. Surg.* (1954) **62**, 591–597.
463. G. D. READ, L'Accouchement naturel. *Bull. Acad. méd., Paris* (1954), 263–276.
464. G. D. READ, *Antenatal Illustrated. The Natural Approach to Happy Motherhood*. Heinemann, London (1957).
465. LA RELAXATION, Société Française de Médecine Psychosomatique —Aspects théoriques et pratiques. Volume published under the auspices of P. ABOULKER, L. CHERTOK and M. SAPIR. *Expansion Scientificque edit.*, Paris 1958.
466. Report of a Subcommittee appointed by the Psychological Medicine Group Committee of the British Med. Ass. on the 'Medical Use of Hypnotism', Suppl. *Brit. Med. J.* (1955), 190–193.
467. Resolution of the *Kiev Congress* (90), 80–84.
468. M. RIVIÈRE and L. CHASTRUSSE, La douleur en obstétrique. *Rev. Franç. Gynéc.* (1954) **49**, 247–276.
469. H. ROBERTS, L. D. P. WOOTEN, K. M. KANE and W. E. HARNETT, The value of antenatal preparation. *J. Obstet. Gynaec., Brit. Emp.* (1953) **60**, 404–408.
470. R. L. ROCHAT, L'accouchement sans douleur. *Praxis* (1955) **44**, 982–984.
471. R. L. ROCHAT and G. ROSSEL, 400 cas d'accouchements sans douleur selon la méthode psychoprophylactique à la maternité Universitaire de Lausanne. *Praxis* (1956) **45**, 1012–1014.
472. H. E. RODWAY, A statistical study on the effects of exercises on childbearing. *J. Obstet. Gynaec. Brit. Emp.*, (1947), **54**, 77–85.
473. J. ROF CARBALLO, *Patologia Psicosomatica*. Paz Montalvo, Madrid (1950).

474. F. L. ROGERS, Dangers in the Read method in patients with major personality problems. *Amer. J. Obstet. Gynec.* (1956), 1236.
475. A. ROLLAND and P. ROLLAND, L'accouchement sans douleur à domicile, à la campagne. *Revue de la Nouvelle Médecine* (1954), 55–64.
476. G. ROSEN, Mesmerism and surgery. A strange chapter in the history of anesthesia. *J. Hist. Med.* (1946), 527–550.
477. R. ROUCHY, Accouchement dirigé. *Ouest Médical, Paris* (1957) **10**, 177–182.
478. P. A. ROUX, *L'Accouchement sans Douleur*. Thesis, Paris (1954).
479. J. ROUX and H. DE WATTEVILLE, Le niveau intellectuel et ses relations avec l'accouchement sans douleur. *Journée d'Études sur les Méthodes Psychologiques en Analgésie Obstétricale, Paris*, 7 April 1957.
480. Th. RUST, Zur psychischen, Prophylaxe des Geburtsschmerzes (über die 'Natürliche Geburt'). *Schweiz. Med. Wschr.* (1953) **83**, 1209–1212.
481. Th. RUST, Zur Prophylaxe der Geburtschwerzes. *Gynecologia* (1956) **142**, 368–372.
482. U. VON RUTTE, Der Einfluss der Schwangerschaftsgymnastik auf den Geburtsschmerz. *Gynaecologia*, (1951) **32**, 274–276.
483. G. M. SALGANNIK, *Leningrad Congress* (76), 65.
484. G. M. SALGANNIK, The origin of the pains of childbirth. *Novosti Meditz.*, Academy of Medical Sciences, Moscow (1952) **30**, 11–19. French abstract. *Cahiers de Méd. Soviétique* (1956) 98–100.
485. G. M. SALGANNIK, *Pain of Childbirth and Analgesia*, Medguiz., Moscow (1953), French transl. Chap. 2, *Commission de Gynéc. Obstet. France—URSS* (1954).
486. SALLIS (DE BADE), Der Hypnotismus in der Geburtshilfe. *Frauenarzt* (1888) 9–42, 72–80.
487. W. SARGENT and R. FRASER, Inducing light hypnosis by hyperventilation. *Lancet* (1938), 778.
488. S. D. SAUNDERS, Accouchement en état magnétique. *J. Magnét.* (1852), 337.
489. H. SAUTER, Behampfung des Geburtsschmerzes. *Schweiz. med. Wschr.* (1956) **86**, 201–204.
490. B. SAWYER, Experiences with labor procedure of Grantly Dick Read, *Amer. J. Obstet. Gynec.* (1946) **51**, 852–858.
491. L. SCHEBAT, De l'accouchement psychoprophylactique médicalement dirigé. *Bull. Féd. Soc. Gyn. Obst., Paris* (1956) **8**, 433–434.
492. P. SCHILDER, *The Image and Appearance of the Human Body*, International University Press, New York (1951).
493. H. SCHIRMACHER, Zur Prophylaxe des Geburtsschmerzes. *Med. Mschr.*, Stuttgart (1956) **10**, 11–16.
494. R. SCHMIEDECK, Zum Problem der schmerzlosen Geburt. *Klin. Med.* (1953) **8**, 449–459.

495. J. M. SCHNECK, Self-hypnosis in obstetrics; case report and comment. *Brit. J. med. Hypnot.* (1952) **2**, 1–3.
496. VON SCHRENCK-NOTZING, Eine Geburt in der Hypnose. *Z. Hypnot.* (1893) **1**, 49–52.
497. J. H. SCHULTZ, *Uebungsheft für das Autogene Training*, 6th ed. Georg Thieme Verlag, Stuttgart (1952).
498. J. H. SCHULTZ, *Das Autogene Training (Konzentrative Selbstenstpannung)* 9th ed., Georg Thieme Verlag, Stuttgart (1956).
499. F. SCHULTZE-RHONHOF, Der hypnotische Geburtsdämmerschlaf. *Zbl. Gynäk.* (1922), 247–257.
500. F. SCHULTZE-RHONHOF, Zum Kapital Hypnosegeburten. *Zbl. Gynäk.* (1923), 476–483.
501. J. SEABRA-DINIS, Accouchement sans douleur? Accouchement sans crainte? Accouchement naturel? *An. portugueses Psiquiat.* (1954) **61**, 94–111.
502. J. SEABRA-DINIS, O parte sem dor por psicoterapie. *J. Méd. Porto* (1954), **23**, 961–964.
503. J. SEABRA-DINIS, Bases cientificas e practicas da psicoprofilaxia das dores do porto. *O. Med. Porto* (1955), **6**,
504. A. B. SEMIANNIKOV, A note on the question of the use of hypnosis in obstetrics. *J. Akouch. i Jenskikh Bolezni* (1907), 58–65.
505. B. SERVICE, Physiotherapy in obstetrics in New Zealand. *Physiotherapy, Lond.* (1955) **41**, 180–182.
506. P. SIMON, L'accouchement sans douleur par la méthode psychoprophylactique. *Bull. méd., Paris* (1955) **69**, 71–76.
507. M. M. SIROTA, A comparative assessment of the psychoprophylactic method and the method of verbal suggestion in obstetrical analgesia. *Akoush. Ginek.* (1956) **1**, 74–75.
508. R. DE SOLDENHOFF, The assessement of relaxation in obstetrics. *Practioner* (1956) **176**, 410–415.
509. S. SOPA *et al.*, Aplicarea metodei extemporanne de psihoprofilaxie e durelilor de nastere. *Obst. ginecol.* (1956) **4**, 240–247.
510. A. A. STEPANOVA, A combined method of psychoprophylactic and medicinal obstetrical analgesia. *Akush Ginek.* (1955) **5**, 75–76.
511. L. STERNWEILER, Natural childbirth. *S. Afr. med. J.* (1956) **30**, 1041–1042.
512. B. STOKVIS, *Hypnose in der Aerzlicher Praxis*. Karger, Bale, (1955).
513. M. STRAKER, Psychological factors during pregnancy and childbirth. *Canad. med. Assoc. J.*, (1954) **70**, 510–514.
514. E. SUPRONOWICZ, Les résultats généraux de l'application de la méthode psychoprophylactique d'accouchement sans douleur. *Ginek. polska* (1956) **6**, 785–789.
515. J. C. SVARTZ, *Résultats Obtensu dans l'Accouchement sans Douleur par la Méthode Psychoprophylactique. Perspectives d'Association a la Méthode de Perfusion Intra-Veineuse de Post-hypophyse.* Thesis, Paris, Faculté de Médecine (1955), No. 1111.
516. SYMPOSIUM: *Brain Mechanisms and Consciousness.* The Council for

International Organisations of Medical Sciences. Blackwell Scientific Publications, Oxford (1954).
517. M. M. SYKRINE, Three years experience in the obstetrical hypnotarium of Kiev. *Pediat Akush. Ginek.* (1950) 28–30.
518. F. A. SYROVATKO and V. I. IAKHONTOV, Changes in the EEG during childbirth. *Akush. Ginek.* (1953), 9–17.
519. F. A. SYROVATKO, Theory and practice in the preparation of pregnant women for childbirth. *Ahouch. i Guin,* Moscow (1957) **4**, 1–7.
520. T. SZASZ, The ego, the body and pain. *J. Amer. Psychoanal. Ass.* (1955) **3**, 177–200.
521. T. SZASZ, *Pain and Pleasure.* Basic Books Inc. Publishers, New York (1957).
522. TATZEL, Eine geburt in der hypnose. *Z. Hypnot.* (1893) **1**, 245–247.
523. A. A. TEREKHOVA, Practice of the psychoprophylactic preparation for childbirth in the obstetrical institutes of the U.S.S.R. *Kiev Congress* (90), 22–28.
524. M. TERRY, *Hidden Wealth and Hiding People.* Putnam, New York (1934).
525. I. TERZI, L'importance des rapports psychomoteurs dans l'accouchement naturel. *La Journée d'Études sur les Méthodes Psychologiques en Analgesie Obstetricale,* Paris 7 April 1957.
526. B. THIS, *Sur une Nouvelle Orientation Médicale: l'Accouchement Psychoprophylactique.* Thesis, Nancy (1954).
527. L. THOMPSON, Attitudes of primiparae as observed in a prenatal clinic. *Ment. Hyg. Concord* (1942) **26**, 243–256.
528. THOMAS, (1) Accouchement normal—Suppression par suggestion des douleurs de dilatation de descente.—Conservation des douleurs terminales concassantes.
 (2) Tentative d'anesthésie par suggestion dans un accouchement.—Insuccès.
 (3) Accouchement laborieux.—Rétrécissement du bassin.—Suppression des douleurs de la contraction utérine, pendant le sommeil provoqué.—Suggestion d'un rythme réguler dans les contractions et de l'anesthésie pendant l'application du forceps. Conservation des douleurs terminales du dégagement de la tête. FONTAN and SÉGARD [164], 302–303.
529. H. THOMS and F. GOODRICH, Training for childbirth. *J. Amer. med. Ass.* (1949), **140**, 1256–1258.
530. H. THOMS, *Training for Childbirth: a Programme of Natural Childbirth with Rooming-in.* McGraw-Hill, New York (1950).
531. H. THOMS, The preparation for childbirth programme. A Commentary. *Obstet. Surv. Baltimore* (1955), **10**.
532. H. THOMS and E. KARLOVSKY, Two thousand deliveries under a training for childbirth program. *Amer. J. Obstet. Gynec.* (1954), **68**, 279–284.

533. H. THOMS, L. ROTH and D. LINTON, *Understanding Natural Childbirth: a book for the expectant mother.* McGraw-Hill, New York. (1950).
534. H. THOMS and R. H. WYATT, One thousand consecutive deliveries under a childbirth program. *Amer. J. Obstet. Gynec.* (1951), 205–209.
535. H. THOMS and E. WIEDENBACH, Comfort during labour. *J. Amer. med. Ass.* (1954) **156**, 3–5.
536. H. THOMS, A wider outlook in obstetrics. *Amer. J. Obstet. Gynec.* (1956) **72**, 1305–1308.
537. H. THOMS and W. C. BILLINGS, A consideration of childbirth programs. *New Engl. J. Med.* (1956) **255**, 860–862.
538. A. A. TOKARSKI, The therapeutic use of hypnotism. *Congress of Russian doctors at Moscow* (1891).
539. R. M. TRUE, Obstetrical hypnoanalgesia. *Amer. J. Obstet. Gynec.* (1954) **67**, 373–376.
540. W. TRUMMLER, Über hypnosegebursten, *Zbl. Gynäk.* (1950) **10**, 585–596.
541. S. TSOULADZE and J. COENCA, Eléments psychophysiologiques de préparation à l'accouchement. *La Journée d'Études sur les Méthodes Psychologiques en Analgésie Obstétricale*, Paris, 7 April 1957.
542. I. T. TSVETKOV, Obstetrical analgesia by direct verbal suggestion without prenatal psychotherapeutic preparation. *Akush. Ginek.* (1941), 32–36.
543. D. H. TUKE, *Illustrations of the Influence of the Mind upon the Body.* London (1872).
544. C. TUPPER, Conditioning for childbirth. *Amer. J. Obstet. Gynec.* (1956) **71**, 733–740.
545. *Twenty years of Nurse-Midwifery, 1933–1953.* Maternity Center Association, New York.
546. B. D. VAN AUKEN and D. K. TOMLINSON, An appraisal of patient training for childbirth. *Amer. J. Obstet. Gynec.* (1953) **66**, 100–105.
547. A. VAN GENNEP, *Manuel du Folklore Français Contemporain.* Vol. 1, ed. Auguste Picard, Paris (1943).
548. F. E. VARCHAVSKAIA, Psychoprophylaxis of the pains of childbirth and the most rational medical treatments. *Soviet. Med.* (1956) **2**, 73–76.
549. VARNIER and SECHEYRON [26], AUVARD and SECHEYRON.
550. VELANDER, Un cas de mutisme mélancolique guéri par suggestion. *Rev. Hypnot, Paris* (1890), 175–176.
551. P. VELLAY and ALINE VELLAY, *Témoignages sur l'Accouchement sans Douleur par la Méthode Psychoprophylactique.* Seuil, Paris (1956).
552. P. VELLAY, Le mot 'sans douleur' est-il justifié? *Bull. Féd. Soc. Gyn. Obstet. Paris*, (1956) **8**, 559–561.
553. I. Z. VELVOVSKI, An attempt to clarify the psychoprophylactic method in painless childbirth using the ideas of I. P. Pavlov. *Leningrad Congress* (89), 41–48.

554. I. Z. VELVOVSKI, Psychoprophylaxis of the pains of childbirth: a complex system. *Pediat. Akush. Ginek.* (1951) **3**, 18–21.
555. I. Z. VELVOVSKI, The principle of the physiological treatment of Pavlov. *Vrach. Dyelo.* (1952).
556. I. Z. VELVOVSKI, La Journée d'Études sur les Méthodes Psychologiques en Analgésie Obstétricale, Paris, 7 April 1957.
557. I. Z. VELVOVSKI, E. A. CHOUGOM and V. A. PLOTITCHER, The psychoprophylactic and psychotherapeutic method in painless childbirth. *Pediat. Akush. Ginek.* (1950).
558. I. Z. VELVOVSKI, K. I. PLATONOV, V. A. PLOTITCHER and E. A. CHOUGOM, *Psychoprophylactic.* Medguiz, Leningrad (1954).
559. I. A. VELVOVSKI, V. A. PLOTITCHER and E. A. CHOUGOM, Obstetrical analgesia. Psychoprophylactic. *Akush. Ginek.* (1950) **6**, 6–12.
560. H. VERMELIN, Le problème actual de l'accouchement. *Rev. méd. Nancy*, (1955) **80**, 12–15.
561. H. VERMOREL, *L'Accouchement sans Douleur par la Méthode Psychoprophylactique à la Lumière de l'Enseignement Physiologique de Pavlov.* Camugli, Lyon, (Bibliographie).
562. L. F. VICENTE, Parto sem dor; metodo psicoprofilactica. Experiencias de un ano no Hospital do Ultramar. *J. Méd. Porto.* (1955) **28**, 5–15.
563. M. V. VIGDOROVITCH, Group suggestion as a method for preparing pregnant women for painless childbirth. *Tezissi dokl. na Il Oukrainskom Siezdie akouch. i Guin.*, Kiev, (1938) 34–46.
564. Y. VITTOZ-MEYNAD, Quelques résultats obtenus par l'association de l'accouchement dirigé et de la méthode psychoprophylactique. *Sem. Hôp.*, Paris, (1956), 3038–3040.
565. A. VOISIN, Un accouchement dans l'état d'hypnotisme. *Rev. Hypnot.* Paris (1896), 360–361.
566. M. VOJTA, Certain problems concerning psychoprophylactic preparation. *Csl. Gynaek.* (1953) **18**, 193–211.
567. M. VOJTA, Some observations on the theoretical basis of the psychoprophylactic method of painless childbirth. *Prakt. Lék. Praha* (1953) **33**, 5–6.
568. F. A. VÖLGYESI, Freud and Pavlov., Proceedings of the meeting at Fribourg *J. Nevropath. i Psikh. Korssakov*, **11** (1957) 1430–5 (Russian).
569. M. VOLLMER, Clinical experiences and observations on the use of relaxation methods in obstetrical practice. *Second Conference* [438] 50–59.
570. P. WALLIN and R. RILEY, Reactions of mothers to pregnancy and adjustment of offspring in infancy. *Amer. J. Orthopsychiat.* (1950) **20**, 616–622.
571. H. DE WATTEVILLE, (3) L'accouchement sans douleur, à Genève.
572. H. DE WATTEVILLE, (3) L'accouchement sans douleur, à Genève, *Med. et Hyg.*, Genève (1956) p. 460.
573. H. DE WATTEVILLE, The use of obstetrical analgesia at the Maternity

Hospital of Genève. *J. Obstet. Gynaec., Brit. Emp.*, (1957) **73**, 473–491.
574. G. DE WERRA and P. DUBUIS, Considérations sur la méthode psychoprophylactique de l'accouchement en clientèle privée. *Praxis*, (1956) **45**, 1014–1016.
575. O. G. WETTERSTRAND, *L'Hypnotisme et ses Applications à la Médecine Pratique*. French Transl: P. Valentin and T. Lindford, O. Doin, Paris (1899).
576. J. DE WIAZEMSKY, Cas d'application de l'hypnotisme contre les douleurs de l'accouchement. *Rev. Hypnot., Psris*, (1908), 80–82.
577. J. WIAZEMSKY, Cas d'application de l'hypnose pendant l'accouchement. Travaux de la Société Physico-Médicale de Saratoff (1904). Quoted by WIAZEMSKY [576].
578. G. VON WOLFF, Des geburtshilfliche Dämmerschlaf in Hypnose, mit besonderer Berücksichtigung seiner Technik. *Archiv. Gynaek.* (1927) **129**, 23–64.
579. E. WOOD, Opération chirurgicale pratiquée dans l'état d'hypnotisme. *Rev. Hypnot., Paris*, (1890), 246–247.
580. R. YMENET, L'Accouchement dit 'sans douleur'. Méthode néo-Pavlovienne. *J. Kinesithérapie* (1954), **3**, 6–8.
581. H. ZAIDMAN, Deux ans de préparation psychoprophylactique à l'accouchement dans les Centres de Santé. *La Journée d'Études sur les Méthodes Psychologiques en Analgésie Obstétricale, Paris*, 7 April 1957.
582. V. I. ZDRAVOMYSLOV, *Experience in the Application of Hypnosis in Obstetrics and in Gynaecology*. Medguiz, Leningrad, (1930).
583. V. I. ZDRAVOMYSLOV, *Hypnosis and Suggestion in Obstetrics and in Gynaecology*. Thesis, Moscow (1938).
584. V. I. ZDRAVOMYSLOV, *Leningrad Congress* (89), p. 68.
585. V. I. ZDRAVOMYSLOV, *Obstetrical Analgesia by Suggestion*. Medguiz, Moscow (1956).
586. E. ZWEIFEL, Über die Schmerzlose Geburt. *Münch. med. Wschr.*, (1922) **2**, 52–53.
587. M. ZWICKER, Suggestion und analgesie. *Münch. med. Wschr.*, (1952) **94**, 737–741.

AUTHOR INDEX

Abbé Faria, 2
Abraham, 87
Airapetiantz, 99
Ajuriaguerra, 84, 161, 162, 212
Ambrose, 87
Amfiteatrov, 49
Angelergues, 94, 151, 156, 158, 164, 182
Anokhine, 100
Arlaud, 167
Arnoldova, 141, 147, 149
Aron, 1
Assatourov, 128, 142
Astakhov, 96, 136
Auken, Van, 6, 7
Auvard, 15, 16
Auzias, 216
Azam, 7

Babinski, 2, 22
Bansillon, 73
Barahona Fernandez, 173
Baux, 165, 177
Beaunis, 14
Bechterew, 30
Belochapko, 98, 105, 113, 129, 134, 138, 147
Berloz, 172
Belozerski, 42
Bermudes, 172
Bernheim, 9, 14, 158
Billings, 66
Birman, 43
Blanchard, 16
Blanche Edwards, 17
Bloos, 199
Bocci, 77
Bojovski, 38
Bonhomme, 178
Bonne, 24
Bonvallet, 101, 188
Bonwill, 16

Boulavintseva, 149
Bourrel, 151, 153, 155, 177, 214
Braid, 2, 6, 8
Brenman, 32, 189
Broca, 7, 8
Brunn, Von, 1
Budin, 15
Burnett, 61
Burger, 84
Burger-Eastman, 86
Burthiault, 167
Buxton, 66
Bykov, 98

Chaigneau, 17
Chapus, 166
Charcot, 14, 19
Chastrusse, 165, 178, 195
Chesnais, de, 17
Chestopal, 32
Chiaudano, 77
Chichkova, 96, 125, 130
Chlifer, 37, 38
Chougom, 56, 125, 145
Choupik, 116, 146
Clark, 87, 89, 91
Coenca, 162, 165, 209
Colette, 151
Corbin, 64
Cotteel, 168
Cramond, 62

Danilevski, 30
Dantec, 165
Daron, 96
Davidenkov, 98, 105
Davidson, 66, 67
Davitti, 77
Deaver, 67
Delay, 20
Dell, 188
Dellepiane, 76
Demangeat, 84

INDEX

Deutsch, 200, 210
De Chesnais, 17
De Grandchamps, 17
De Jong, 18
De Lee, 9, 67, 87
De Leeuwe, 169
De Puysegur, 2
De Watteville, 170
Diaz, 9
Dietlin, 165
Dobbin, 180
Dobrovolsky, 17, 30
Doline, 109
Doniguevitch, 33, 92, 113
Donovan, 209
Dos Santos, 172
Draps, 169
Du Potet, 4, 11
Dubois, 36, 158
Dubuis, 167, 172
Dumontpallier, 15, 17, 26
Duncan, 67

Ebner, 61
Economides, 94, 152, 160, 216
Egron, 72, 205
Eligulachvili, 103, 197
Elliotson, 5
Eps, Van, 70, 179
Erofeeva, 99
Esdaile, 5

Falk, 24
Fanton, 17
Faria, Abbé, 2
Favarel, 166
Fere, 15
Ferenczi, 20
Ferguson, 193
Ferrier, 177
Floel, 18, 24, 28
Foi, 113, 129, 134, 138
Foissac, 11
Fodor, 201
Follin, 7
Ford, 193
Forel, 9
Fort, 9

Fraipont, 17
Franke, 28
Freed, 87
Freedman, 79, 193, 217
Friedlander, 24
Friedman, 65
Frigyesi, 24
Freud, 19, 185, 198
Fromm-Reichmann, 190
Gaillard, 165
Garmacheva, 96
Garnier, 167
Gavel, 168
Gellhorn, 101
Geisendorf, 170
Gill, 32
Glasner, 1
Goirand, 166
Goodrich, 53, 63
Gomez, 77
Gourvitch, 186
Grandchamps, de, 17
Grandaliano-Mollard, 167
Green, 87
Greenacre, 202
Gregoire, 168
Gueckel, 24
Gueorguievski, 39
Guerenstein, 35
Guerineau, 8
Guillain, 19
Guze, 87, 91

Haddon, 192
Hall, 63
Hallauer, 24
Hardy, 79
Harlin, 72
Heardman, 53, 59, 61
Heberer, 24, 26
Held, 209
Hellmann, 75, 148, 215
Heron, 87
Hogan, 67
Hrdlicka, 192
Hugelin, 101, 186
Husson, 11

INDEX

IAKHONTOV, 149
IAKOVLEV, 135
IVANOV, 125, 130
IVANOV-SMOLENSKI, 98

JACOBSON, 56, 207
JANET, 22, 158
JAVERT, 79
JEANSON, 151, 165
JELOKHOVTSEVA, 148
JIMENEZ, 173, 214
JOIRE, 18, 28
JONG, DE, 18
JORDANIA, 98, 106, 138, 140
JOURNEE, 17

KALACHNIK, 36
KARLOVSKY, 64
KARTCHNER, 202
KATCHAN, 42
KEKTCHEEV, 99
KHETCHINACHVILI, 148
KINGSBURY, 17
KIRITCHENKO, 113, 120, 122
KIRSTEIN, 24, 27
KLEIN, 201
KLEMPERER, 34
KLINE, 87–91
KLOOSTERMAN, 70
KOGANOV, 46, 129
KOGERER, 24, 26
KONSTANTINOV, 98, 106, 112
KOPIL-LEVINA, 40
KORABELNIK, 96
KROENIG, 24
KROGER, 9, 59, 77, 87, 89, 90

LACOMME, 176
LAFONTAINE, 12, 176
LAIRD, 67
LAMAZE, 151, 156, 164, 175, 179, 214
LANGEVIN-DROGUET, 71
LANDISBERG, 209
LARREY, 7

LARRIBERE, 165
LE LORIER, 166
LEE, 16
LE MENANT DE CHESNAIS, 17
LEE, DE, 9, 67, 87
LEEUWE, DE, 169
LEPAGE, 71
LEVIT, 135, 138
LICHTSCHEIN, 18
LIEBAULT, 2, 8, 12, 13, 14, 176
LIEGEOIS, 9, 14
LOHMER, 76
LOURIE, 115
LOYSEL, 6
LUGEOL, 17
LUKAS, 75
LUYS, 17
LYONNET, 178

MABILLIE, 9
MADDERS, 61
MAGOUN, 100
MALAGUTI, 165
MALCOVATI, 173
MANDY, 59, 77, 78
MANSFELD, 24
MARTIUS, 76
MASON, 9
MATVEEV, 17, 30
MAUREL, 165
MAYER, 70, 178
MEAD, 192
MEDEIROS, 172
MERZ, 75
MESMER, 1
MESNET, 9, 15
MEYLAN, 172
MICHAEL, 87, 88, 207
MIEVILLE, 75
MILLER, 67
MOLONEY, 218
MONJARDINO, 172
MONTGOMERY, 61
MORUZZI, 100
MULDVORF, 163, 164
MURPHY, 68, 101, 215

INDEX

Nassauer, 23
Newbold, 87
Nicolaev, 32, 33, 42, 94, 101, 109, 111, 113, 131, 135, 181
Nikouline, 148
Nixon, 60
Nogueira, 77
Nordmann, 171
Notter, 72, 73, 162, 205

Oettingen, von, 24
Ogoulbostan-Essenova, 192

Pavlov, 21, 98, 111
Pchonik, 100
Peeters, 169
Petit, 16
Petrov-Maslakov, 98, 106, 113, 135
Pigeaud, 73
Pinoli, 77
Pitres, 9
Platonov, 21, 30, 39, 40, 94
Plotitcher, 48, 110, 154, 200
Porak, 15
Portnuff, 70
Postolnik, 36
Potet, du, 4, 11
Preissman, 192
Prill, 76, 84
Pritzl, 15
Prudent, 165
Puysegur, de, 2

Quichon, 167

Rabinovitch, 135, 138
Raimbault, 70
Ramadier, 9
Ramon Cajal, 18
Ransom, 60, 215
Rapaport, 190
Ravina, 165
Razdolski, 96
Redlich, 217
Rivière, 165, 178, 195
Roberts, 60

Rochat, 171
Rodway, 79
Roelens, 94, 156
Rof-Carballo, 184
Rogers, 68
Rolland, 166
Rosen, 1
Rouchy, 168
Roux, 165
Rutte, von, 74

Salgannik, 95, 104, 109, 113
Sallis, 17
Santos, dos, 172
Sargent, 16
Sauter, 75
Sawyer, 64
Schebat, 167
Schirmacher, 76
Schmiedeck, 76
Schneck, 87
Schoenholz, 24
Schrenk-Notzing, 17
Schultz, 82, 207
Schultze-Rhonhof, 24, 25
Schoysman, 169
Seabra-Dinis, 172
Setchenov, 15, 16, 17
Semiannikov, 30
Service, 63
Sirota, 129, 142
Soldenhof, 60
Stepanova, 134
Sternweiler, 63
Stokvis, 16
Straker, 202
Svartz, 165
Syrkine, 46
Syrovatko, 99, 148, 149
Szasz, 199

Tatzel, 000
Terekhova, 143, 148, 149
Terry, 192
Terzi, 77
This, 165
Thomas, 15

INDEX

Thoms, 53, 64, 215
Tokarski, 30
Tomlinson, 67
Tourevski, 38
True, 87
Trummler, 28
Tsouladze, 162, 209
Tsvetkov, 40
Tuke, 201
Tuke, Hack, 6, 201
Tupper, 68

Van Auken, 67
Van Eps, 70, 179
Varchavskaia, 135, 143, 146
Velander, 9
Vellay, 151, 175, 179, 214
Velvovski, 32, 49, 94, 97, 102, 113, 179
Vermorel, 94, 152, 159, 163, 216
Vicente, 172
Vigdorovitch, 46
Vittoz-Meynard, 167

Voisin, 17
Vollmer, 88, 215
Von Brunn, 1
Von Oettingen, 24
Von Rutte, 74
Von Wolff, 28

Watteville, de, 170
Werra, 167, 172
Wetterstrand, 17
Wiazemsky, 17, 20
Wiedenbach, 215
Wolff, von, 28
Wood, 9
Wyatt, 64

Ymenet, 165

Zaidman, 168
Zatchepitski, 113
Zdravomyslov, 39, 47, 98, 109, 134
Zweifel, 24

SUBJECT INDEX

Abdominal effleurage, 121
Abdominal massage, 15
Amnesia and hypnosis, 80
Analgesia, 1
   and behaviour, 216
   and psychotherapy, 1
   in the Bible, 1
Analgesiant factors, 204
Analgesic effect, 000
   by action on anxiety, 211
Animal magnetism, 2, 5
Ante-natal exercises, 56
Anxiety, 211
Artificial hysteria, 19
Astakhov test for suggestibility, 43
Autogenous training, 82, 86
Autohypnosis, 134

Birman test for suggestibility, 43
Breathing, 57, 74

Cardiovascular affections, 130
Cartoons, use of, 77
Childbirth,
   conduct of in hypnosuggestive method, 90
   in primitive societies, 192
Colours, use of, 76
Conditioned reflexes, 21, 98
Cortex, 21, 99
   role in perception of pain, 99
   state of during childbirth, 106
Cortical activation, 107
'Couvade', 215

Didactic elements in Prill method, 86
Didactic factor in psychological analgesia, 204
Dilatation, 154
Direct suggestion, 40

Doctor-patient relationship, 38, 39
Dolorimeter, 79

Educated childbirth, 66
Education and suggestion, 161
Electroneuromyometer, 82
Episiotomy, 87, 91
Exercises, 155, 205

Fear, 55, 114, 198, 211
   suppression of, 119
   origin of, 200
Films, use of, 77
Forceps, use of, 69, 74, 76, 87, 145, 172

Gramophone, use in conduct of childbirth, 90

Hebrews, 1
Higher nervous activity, 120
Husband, participation of, 214
Hypnoid phases, 21
Hypnonarcosis, 24
Hypnosis, 19, 134
Hypnosuggestive methods, 23, 160
   in Anglo-Saxon countries, 87
   in Germany, 23
   in obstetrics, 15
   in Russia, 30
   mass application of, 46
   results of, 16
   technique of, 15
Hypnotarium, 46
Hypnotic anaesthesia, 5, 21
Hypnotism, 2
Hypnotizability, assessment of, 43

Indirect suggestion, 41, 48
Induction, technique of, 87
Inhibition, 156
Initial interview, 38
Interpersonal relationship, 161, 209

INDEX

Lactation, 127
Lumbar massage, 15, 57
Lumbar pain, 167
Luminous passes, 34

Magnetic anaesthesia, 3, 4
Magnetic analgesia, 5
Masochism, 210
Mental hygiene, 218
Mesmeric passes, 34
Midwife, role in psychoprophylactic method, 115
Motivated suggestion, 41
Muscular release, 177
Music, use of, 76

Narcohypnosis, 28
Nervous types, 112, 131, 166, 188
   case history, 136
   study of, 118, 136
   study of suggestibility, 137
Neuromuscular education, 154
Nomenclature, 152

Obstetrical analgesia,
   method of selection for, 42
   suggestive method, 42
Oxyhaemoglobimeter, 149

Pain, 75, 76, 162, 184, 202
   and anxiety, 198
   degrees of, 145
   emotional factors, 197
   in the Bible, 210
   levels of, 203
   nature of in childbirth, 102
   psychogenic, 103
   real, 47
   reflex-conditioned, 48
   somatic, 103
   suggested, 48
Pain reducing procedure, 121
Pain sensitivity, 103
Painless childbirth,
   advantages, 218
   in civilized society, 191
Parturition, in animals, 195

Pavlovian school, 21
Persuasion, 158
Physical exercises, in autogenous training, 84
Physiotherapetuic factor, 205
Plethysmograph, 138, 148, 150
Posthypnotic suggestion, 26
Pre-eclamptic toxaemia, 130
Prenatal exercises, 61
Preparation, psychosomatic aspects, 67
   in hypnosuggestive methods, 88
Psychoanalytic concepts, 91
'Psycho-infection', 127
Psychological analgesia, 187
   in obstetrics, 204
Psychoprophylactic Method, 47
   application in France, 151
   application in Italy, 173
   application in Spain, 173
   causes of failure, 127
   conduct during, 126
   controversial problems in, 102
   extemporary methods, 128
   in the Soviet Union, 92
   medical and obstetrical advantages, 145
   mistakes during preparation, 124
   personnel employed in, 114, 153
   principles, 98
   psychophysiological studies, 148
   results, 138, 163
   role of speech, 102
   role of suggestion, 110
   theoretical aspects, 97
   with drug induced analgesia, 134
Psychotherapeutic factor, 208
Pulmonary tuberculosis, births amongst patients, 72

Rational psychotherapy, 41
Read method, 53
   applications, 59
   comparison with Velvovski method, 175
   criticism of, 77
   practice, 56

Relaxation, 205
  in autogenous training, 84
  in psychoprophylactic method, 123
  in Read method, 56, 72
Relaxation-rest, 131
Respiratory exercises, 57, 205
  in autogenous training, 84
Rhythmic activity, in autogenous training, 84
R.875, 169

Sleep, 21
Speech, 51, 102, 163, 187
Spirometry, 74
Suggestion, 57, 159

Telephone, use in conduct of childbirth, 90
Thalamus, 42, 55
Tokodynamometer, 49
Toxaemia, 47

Uterine contraction, 75

Velvovski method, comparison with Read, 75

War neuroses, 22

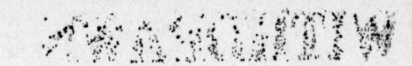